Main

CURE
BACK
PAIN

D0536429

CURE
BACK
PAIN

PERSONALIZED EASY EXERCISES
for Spinal Training to Improve Posture,
Eliminate Tension & Reduce Stress

Jean-François Harvey,
BSc, DO

Robert
ROSE

For complete cataloguing information, see page 256.

Disclaimer
This book is a general guide only and should never be a substitute for the skill, knowledge, and
experience of a qualified medical professional dealing with the facts, circumstances, and symptoms
of a particular case.

The nutritional, medical, and health information presented in this book is based on the research,
training, and professional experience of the author, and is true and complete to the best of his
knowledge. However, this book is intended only as an informative guide for those wishing to know
more about health, nutrition, and medicine; it is not intended to replace or countermand the advice
given by the reader's personal physician. Because each person and situation is unique, the author
and the publisher urge the reader to check with a qualified health-care professional before using any
procedure where there is a question as to its appropriateness. A physician should be consulted before
beginning any exercise program. The author and the publisher are not responsible for any adverse
effects or consequences resulting from the use of the information in this book. It is the responsibility
of the reader to consult a physician or other qualified health-care professional regarding his or her
personal care.

Editor/Copyeditor: Fina Scroppo
Translator: Donna Vekteris
Indexer: Gillian Watts

Design and Production: PageWave Graphics Inc.
    Page layout adapted from *L'Entraînement Spinal*, designed by Christine Hébert
Infographics: Marie-Josée Lalonde
Ambiance Photography: Mathieu Dupuis
Cover and Exercise Photography: Tango
Illustrations: Chantale Boulianne
Anatomical Illustrations: Mathieu Bélanger

The publisher gratefully acknowledges the financial support of our publishing program by the
Government of Canada through the Canada Book Fund.

Published by Robert Rose Inc.
120 Eglinton Avenue East, Suite 800, Toronto, Ontario, Canada M4P 1E2
Tel: (416) 322-6552 Fax: (416) 322-6936
www.robertrose.ca

Printed and bound in Canada

1 2 3 4 5 6 7 8 9 TCP 24 23 22 21 20 19 18 17 16

In memory of Jean-Philippe

Contents

Foreword

"Life is nothing but movement."

— Montaigne

The spinal column, which is the body's true central axis, is amazingly complex. Our back is at the center of our body in our most elaborate movements as well as our most stable postures. Unfortunately, our back is too often the source of pain and discomfort. This book is designed to help you better understand this complexity and get your back moving again in the right away.

For 25 years, I've been experimenting with the different effects of physical training on the back. The back pain I experienced early on in life quickly made me aware of the fact that the back has limitations. First, as an athlete, I noticed since adolescence that playing sports intensively could have a negative impact on the back. At that age I was already wondering what I could do to help my back. Later on, as a sports trainer, I put athletes through extreme routines to strengthen their abdominals and back — routines that were based on the physical fitness trends of that era. Looking back, I think that the majority of these exercises were downright harmful to the back.

In my quest to understand human movement, I studied kinesiology (the science of movement). At the end of these studies, I was in charge of a rehabilitation clinic in the area of workplace accidents, which most often included back injuries. Through trial and error, I learned how

Spinal Training Exercise is Key

June 20, 2002, 10:29 a.m. I'm lying on the patio of the second floor. But there's a problem: I live on the third floor. An ambulance ride to the hospital and a battery of tests follow, and then I am told: "Mr. Latendresse, you have a fractured spinal column. We need to perform emergency surgery on you."

A few days after the operation, the surgeon fills me in on the situation. "Your spinal cord was damaged and I had to fuse three of your vertebrae together. From what we've observed in the last few days, you'll be able to walk again, but we can't predict your percentage of recovery."

Jean-François said: "I can't predict your percentage of recovery but if you're motivated, we'll set a goal for complete recovery. The osteopathy and the choice of exercises will be my responsibility. You'll have the more difficult job. First, you'll have to strengthen your muscles and become as flexible as possible. Your biggest challenge, however, will be to make these exercises part of daily life if you want to hold on to the gains you'll have made during recovery." I was sentenced to getting into shape.

Since 2005, I've been in excellent physical condition. I still do my series of exercises two or three times a week. Two or three times 45 minutes is very little effort to maintain one's quality of life.

But you don't have to wait for an accident before taking charge of your health. Build an exercise program that suits your needs, and most of all, stick with it. Perseverance is the key to good physical condition — for life.

Thank you, Jean-François, for giving me this key.

— R. Latendresse (Patient)

to choose suitable exercises and properly teach patients who were often barely aware of their body. It was primarily two discoveries that would modify my practice. First, I noticed that physical training helps to ease pain and can also resolve back problems, even severe ones. My team often finds solutions to problems that other physical therapists have struggled to uncover. More than 20 years ago, the approach to treating back problems was rest and immobilization, but after seeing the effects of this regimen, it's no surprise that many therapists now advocate the opposite, with physical activity being the first line of defense. Second, I realized that we were not very knowledgeable about back-related issues. Compared to the world of nutrition, which has greatly evolved over the past few decades, the world of physical training has remained at the era of microwave cooking in the 1980s. It may have changed a lot, but the latest knowledge is shared by very few.

Realizing that I lacked the tools to help my patients, I conducted several studies in osteopathy (manual alternative medicine) and completed a thesis on posture. A more rounded understanding of the body allows me to better help my patients. Any regimen, however, would not be complete, without physical activity. In my practice, I consider physical activity as the base on which health is built. Getting the body to move again is the first objective. This principle is at the heart of what I teach my students in my biomechanics courses. (Biomechanics is the science that studies body movement.) A person who does not move will develop problems, and it is the back that is most often affected.

As an osteopath, I do my best to help my patients and I feel gratified each time one of them shows improvement in their health. At the same time, I am conscious of the fact that I am just one element of support in that patient's personal journey. No physical therapist can perform miracles or has the power to change another person's life. It's the patient that needs to take the initiative. The true power of healing lies within us and it is up to us to harness.

Why write this book now? I had often been asked by patients, students, friends and athletes to recommend a good back exercise book. I couldn't find one that suited the needs of patients. These types of books exist only for health-care professionals or are centered on methods or exercise regimens that are currently in vogue, such as yoga or Pilates. This book is my response to this need.

My exercise system, called Spinal Training, is based on a number of exercise methods that have been developed (Pilates, yoga, advanced stretching, rehabilitation exercises, qigong, breathing exercises), as well as the principles of osteopathy, biomechanics and the Godelieve Denys-Struyf (GDS) method, to name a few of the main influences.

Some of the elements in these methods and principles are intertwined and complementary, which makes the book unique. Spinal Training does not purport to be a miracle method, but after years of development and experimentation, it is by far the best contribution that my team and I have made to help people whose goal is to have a healthier back. The exercises illustrated in this book have been tested by many people, both with and without back problems, over a long period of time at my clinic and my training studio.

After reading this book, you will never look at your back in quite the same way, and you will be equipped with some very effective and safe tools to help you. Whether you have lower back pain and are not very active, or an athlete wishing to improve the condition of your back, this book is for you.

Godelieve Denys-Struyf (GDS) is a complex method to stabilize the spine that combines a number of therapies, including stretching poses, manual massage therapy, reflex techniques and stimulation of various muscle groups such as the diaphragm.

Introduction

As an osteopath, I've noted that my patients with back pain have often tried certain exercises to resolve their problem. Sometimes they are successful, but unfortunately, too often they are not. When an exercise program fails, it often results in people giving up the program and all other types of physical training as well. They are then led to believe that they must resort to medication or visit a physical therapist to ease the pain. People who suffer from back pain then lose their autonomy in terms of dealing with the problem, which is a problem in itself.

Even if anti-inflammatory medications diminish their pain (although without healing the underlying condition), and even if a physical therapist is of great help, it's still essential that people maintain as much autonomy as possible when it comes to managing their health. This applies to health in general as well as the back. The foundation of health and life is movement, and a moving back is a healthy back. If that is the case, however, then why do so many people injure themselves exercising?

To answer this question, let's consider the case of a 39-year-old man we will call Aldo who has suffered from back pain for 10 years.

It's January 1st. A new year and new resolutions. At the top of the list, Aldo wants to do something to ease his persistent back pain. Knowing that he needs to strengthen his abdominal muscles to have a good back, Aldo starts with a set of 30 sit-ups a day. He increases them gradually, progressing so well that by the end of the month, he is up to two sets of 75 sit-ups a day. At the end of six weeks, he still has back pain, and even more pain after doing his sit-ups, so he quits. Much to his regret, he does not yet have the sculpted abs of a movie star.

As we will see later, sit-ups are far from the best exercise for the back. They can even be downright harmful! The myth of strong abdominals for a good back still persists today.

The following January 1st rolls around, ushering a new decade for Aldo, who has put on almost 9 pounds and still has backaches. He decides to take matters in his own hands by joining a gym and hiring a personal trainer. The trainer claims that Aldo's back problem is due to weakness in his back muscles. Aldo is given a program to follow that will strengthen the superficial muscles of his back. The program mainly consists of exercises on machines. At the end of five weeks, Aldo quits. His pains have worsened and extend down his right buttock.

It is completely erroneous to think that strengthening the superficial muscles of the back will resolve a back problem. First of all, the priority is to stretch these muscles. As we will see later in the book, the emphasis needs to be placed on the deep muscles of the back, which many people don't know about. You will soon have the pleasure of being introduced to these muscles.

Another year goes by, and Aldo's girlfriend convinces him to start taking yoga, assuring him that it will do him a world of good. All of

> The foundation of health and life is movement, and a moving back is a healthy back. If that is the case, however, then why do so many people injure themselves exercising?

Hollywood is praising its virtues, it's the most "in" thing to do, and now it's time for Aldo to jump on the bandwagon. The only hitch: his girlfriend is extremely flexible and has never had a back problem. As for Aldo, he can barely perform the "sun salutation" that starts off the session and is considered a warm-up. Because his back hurts for two days after each yoga session, he thinks this must be a good sign. But during the eighth session, while he is adopting a posture that involves twisting the back (leaning forward with the torso turned sideways), he feels a sharp pain at the base of his spine. The following day, he wakes up nearly paralyzed, and then hobbles in pain and misery to his doctor, who prescribes anti-inflammatories.

Yoga is a richly complex method that can greatly benefit the body and spirit. However, its practice, in the way it has evolved, calls for a high degree of physical skill as well as a top-notch instructor. For a person who is not guided properly or in tune with their body's limitations, certain yoga exercises are actually dangerous for the back.

Another years rolls around and Aldo adds up the previous year's back-treatment expenses — for osteopathy, acupuncture, massotherapy, kinesitherapy, anti-inflammatory medication, pain relievers, muscle relaxants, a device for toning abdominal muscles electronically, orthopedic soles, etc. The list is long and the bill is high. He thinks he should really go see this trainer who was recommended to him — apparently, she healed her herniated disk by doing 100 bridge exercises a day, and now she is teaching this to people with back problems.

We could go on like this forever, but let's end Aldo's story here. It's a good illustration of two important points: Most people don't know what their back really needs and the exercises they do often don't meet these needs. As we will read later, certain popular exercises even run contrary to these needs. Let's hope that this book will end up in Aldo's hands.

In the following pages, you will learn why, among other things...

- The latest ab super machine will not change your life.
- The force of gravity does not explain back problems.
- Doing sit-ups can be harmful to the back.
- Strengthening superficial back muscles is not very useful.
- Some muscles must be stretched and others strengthened.
- Stretching is not recommended for everybody.
- Intense mat exercises alone are not sufficient for the back.
- Exercise is more effective for the back than medication.
- The spinal column is of prime importance for any activity.
- Backaches affect so many people.
- The body naturally strives to be healthy, not unhealthy.
- A digestive problem can cause backaches.
- The back is directly linked to the nervous system.
- Emotional stress can have an impact on the back.

You will also discover how to…

- have very effective core muscles;
- have good, attractive posture, effortlessly;
- release muscle tension in your back;
- move efficiently and in a fluid way;
- diminish back pain.

How to Use This Book

This book is divided into two parts. The first part (Chapters 1 to 5) is designed to provide you with easy-to-follow information about everything you need to know about your back. After reading this book, you will have a new regard for your back, its anatomy, causes of back pain, diagnoses, proper posture, the body's regulatory systems and effective exercises and the keys to a successful training program.

The second part (Chapters 6 and 7) reads like a cookbook and consists of a step-by-step exercise program. You will find 80 exercises (recipes) and 35 routines (menus) that will answer many different needs. This program has been tested on thousands of people and proven to help you in your quest for a healthy back. What's best, you don't need to integrate all of the 80 exercises in your daily routine for success.

In this program, you will find a routine that best suits you and can be easily modified. As many people can testify, even a little Spinal Training routine is enough to produce big results.

WARNING

Before starting any exercise program, especially a new one, it is recommended that you consult a doctor. If you have back pain, it is essential that you get a medical opinion before jumping into a new activity. Tell your doctor if you intend to take charge of your back by following Spinal Training or any other training.

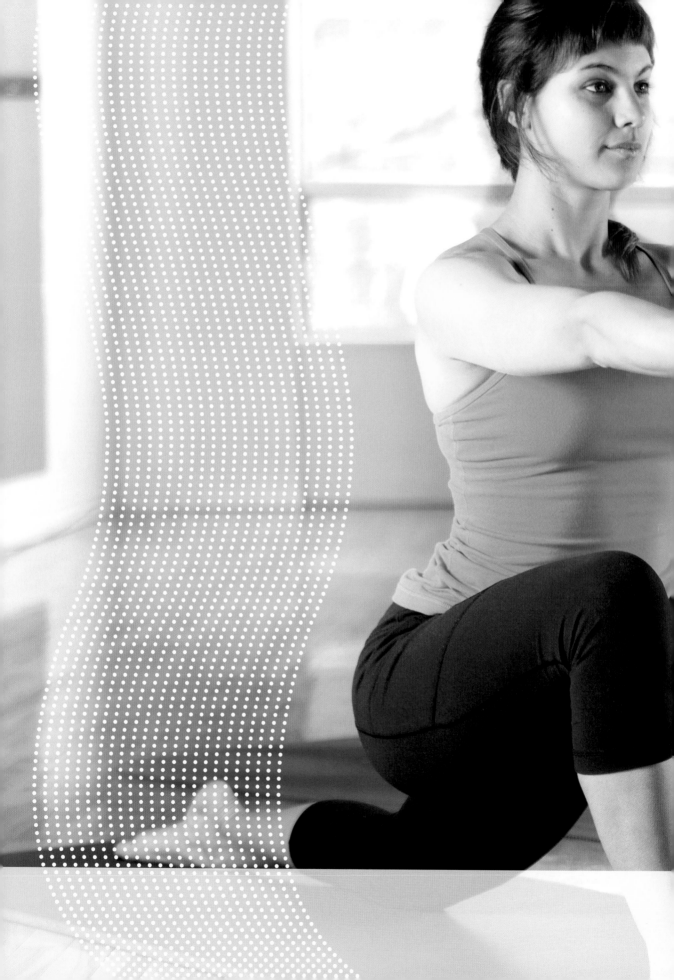

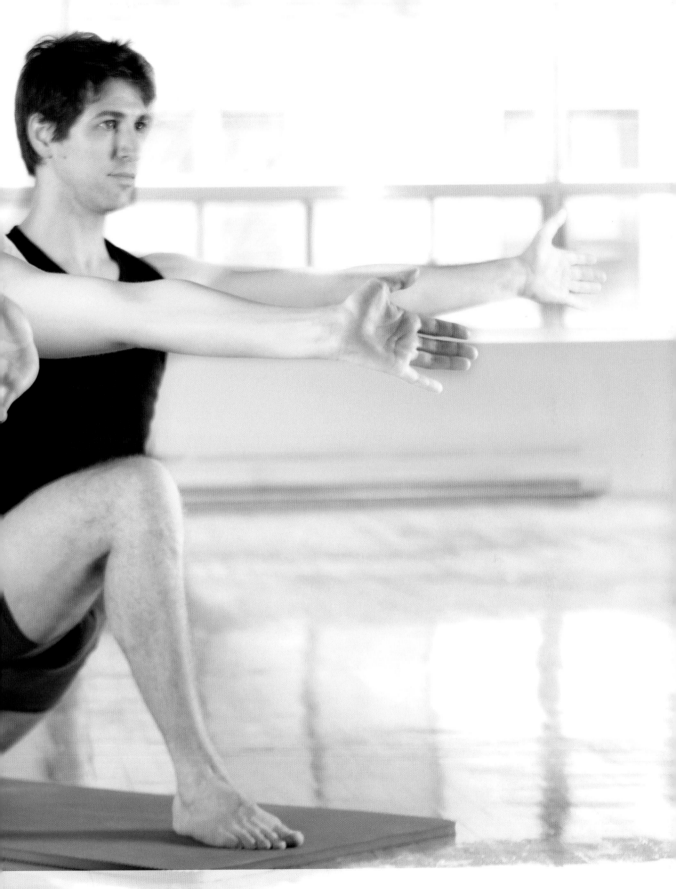

CHAPTER 1: A MAN AND HIS BACK

The Curse of the Century

You're not the only one with a back that isn't working as well as it could. Declared the curse of the 21st century, and already champion of the previous century, it appears that the backache has made a place for itself in our society and is here to stay. All the more reason to question and react rather than be fatalistic. The first question that we can ask ourselves is simple: Why does our back hurt?

Evolution in Brief

Looking at the evolution of the species, it seems obvious that lifestyles have changed considerably since prehistoric times — 3.8 billion years ago — when the only living species, bacteria, were swimming naively in a mixture of methane, ammonia and hydrogen sulfide. It took no less than 3.3 billion years for the first vertebrates to appear, in the form of fish, and the spinal column was born. Leaving an aquatic environment for the promised land 110 million years later, this species developed reptilian feet at the same time as the ability to move in new ways. The spinal column reached its peak in terms of size during the Mesozoic (dinosaur) era. According to the most recent estimates, the spinal column of *Amphicoelias* measured up to 180 feet (55 meters) in length. In comparison, the spinal column of modern man measures about 3 feet (1 meter) in length.

Finally reaching the biped stage (340 million years later!), man developed spectacular skill in walking and running. His body and its spinal column became a superb machine for getting around and moving, giving him a distinct advantage over other species. The very recent arrival of the modern era, urbanization and technological development, however, rapidly changed our way of living, with manual labor giving way to knowledge-based labor. The computer has recently played a dominant role in industrialized societies, which has consequently reduced our level of physical activity in a draconian fashion. A large portion of Earth's inhabitants is now more sedentary than ever. According to the World Health Organization, more than 60% of the population does not achieve the recommended level of physical activity for good health. And the proportion is growing each year.

> A large portion of Earth's inhabitants are now more sedentary than ever.

Evolution

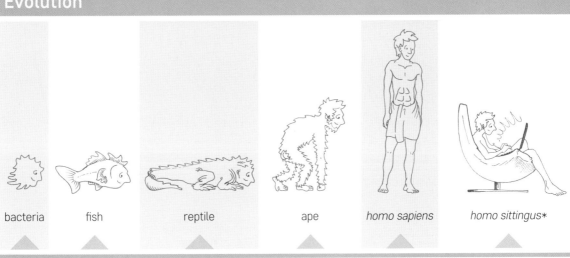

| bacteria | fish | reptile | ape | *homo sapiens* | *homo sittingus*∗ |

∗ See the illustration of "*homo sittingus*" on page 18.

Hours and hours spent in front of a screen:

- The average North American consumer spends 60 hours a week consuming content across different electronic devices.
- Computer users spend about 22 hours a week on their PCs beyond their time spent on computers at work.
- Consumers with tablets use their device for about an hour and 15 minutes daily.
- North Americans are now spending a total of 35 hours a week on the Internet or watching television. The latest statistics also show that Internet usage and TV watching continues to increase every year.

If we add these impressive figures to the number of hours spent sitting at work (increasingly in front of a computer), eating or just simply sitting, and to the number of hours spent lying down, there remains very little time spent in a standing position or in motion.

A New Model of Hominid

In light of this reorganization of our existence to the seated (and collapsed) position, I propose (unofficially) a new model of hominid: *homo sittingus* (seated man).

Homo Sittingus — In His Natural Environment

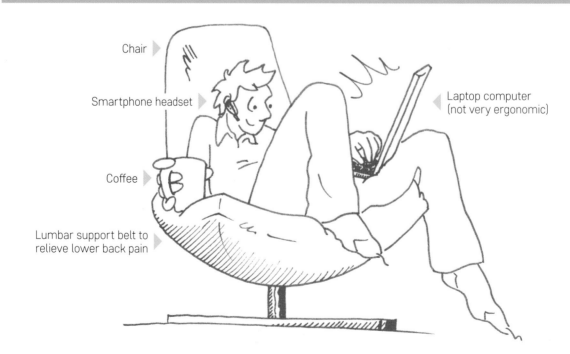

Chair

Smartphone headset

Coffee

Lumbar support belt to relieve lower back pain

Laptop computer (not very ergonomic)

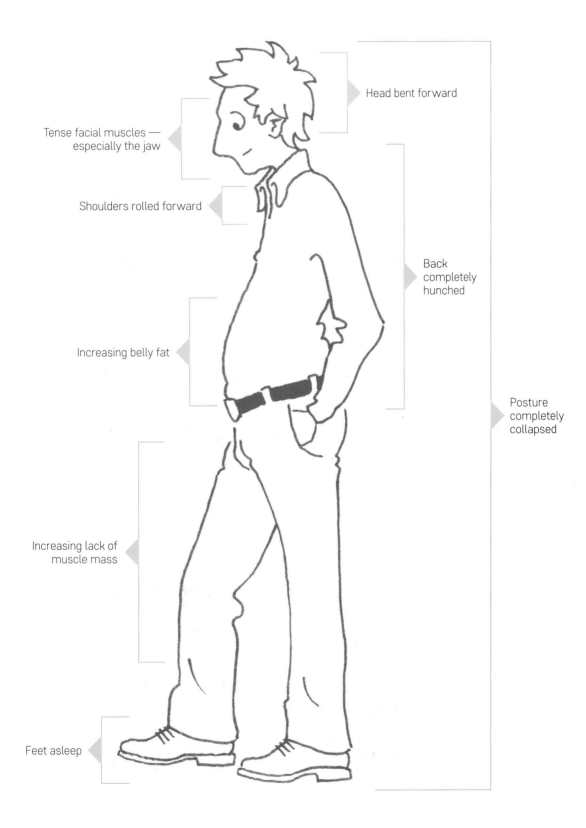

Head bent forward

Tense facial muscles — especially the jaw

Shoulders rolled forward

Back completely hunched

Increasing belly fat

Posture completely collapsed

Increasing lack of muscle mass

Feet asleep

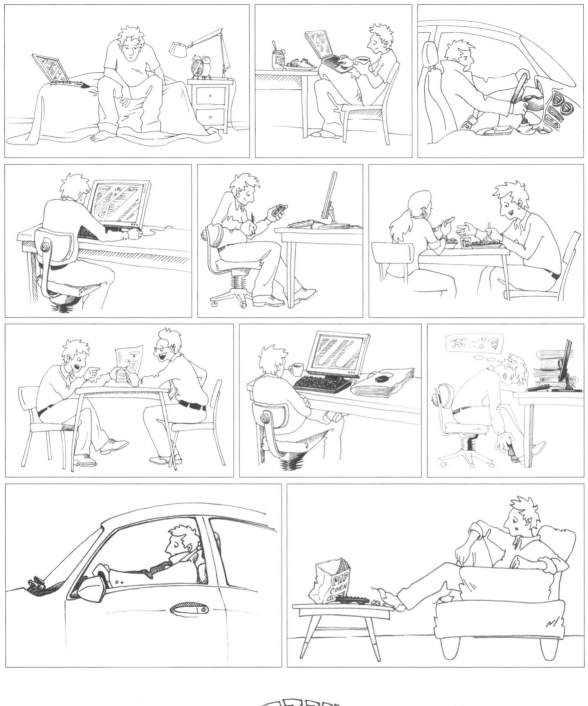

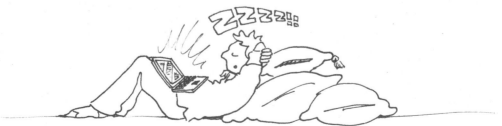

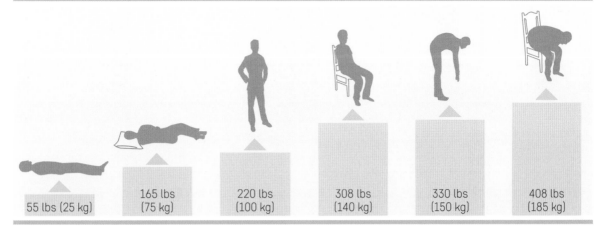

| 55 lbs (25 kg) | 165 lbs (75 kg) | 220 lbs (100 kg) | 308 lbs (140 kg) | 330 lbs (150 kg) | 408 lbs (185 kg) |

Pressure exerted on the disks according to the position.

Homo sittingus is especially present in industrialized societies. He is fond of new technologies. Having a highly developed social network, he spends a great deal of time communicating on Facebook, Twitter, Instagram and other social media in a seated position. He mainly eats processed foods and drinks a lot of coffee to maintain a certain level of energy. Naturally, his back hurts from time to time. When he really thinks about it, his back bothers him more and more with each passing year.

A number of studies have shown that the sitting position puts more pressure on the disks than the standing position or even walking. This explains why people who are struggling with disk problems (for example, degenerative disk disease) more often experience pain when sitting and get relief when standing. To reduce this pressure, the key is to lengthen the spinal column and activate the core muscles of the back.

> When we study the body — how it functions and its movements — we realize that it is clearly adapted to moving, walking, dancing and running, and not to remaining seated in front of a screen.

Inactivity on Trial?

So should we put the blame on inactivity? It seems that we can, for the most part. I'm tempted to say that the real curse of the century is not backache but inactivity. At the same time, you might be asking whether our more active ancestors had back problems. It's a question that is difficult to answer, since there isn't any research that has accurately demonstrated the extent of back problems in our forebears.

One thing is certain, however: When we study the body — the way it works and moves — we realize that it is clearly adapted to moving, walking, dancing and running, and not to remaining seated in front of a screen. The problem is quite complex, however, and many other causes may be at the root of backaches, as you will soon discover in the pages to come.

Are We Subjected to Gravity?

You've probably heard the myth that a backache is simply the result of our bodies being subjected to gravity. Gravity, or gravitational force, is not the problem, but rather a power that is essential to life. It is partly because of gravity that we are equipped with a back of such incredible complexity. Gravitational force pulls us toward everything that surrounds us. The greater the mass of an element, the more we are attracted to it. And because the Earth beneath our feet has a mass of about 5.97 kg x 10^{24} kg — infinitely greater than our own — we are strongly pulled toward its center.

Are we necessarily condemned to collapse on the ground? Newton (who was at the origin of gravitational theory) said no, because all force corresponds to an opposing force of reaction of equal intensity and in the opposing direction. In practical terms, the gravitational force that pulls us toward the ground corresponds to a force of reaction that pushes us off the ground and pulls us toward the sky.

Anatomy of the Back

Before we proceed, here's a closer look at the human anatomy that includes the spinal column and major back muscles. You will be introduced to an amazing structure featuring architecture that defies all the laws of physics and gain a better understanding of the functions that relate to this structure.

What is the Spinal Column For?

The spinal column has three functions:

- to protect the nervous system (the spinal cord and the nerve roots);
- to stabilize the body in space (like the mast of a sailing ship);
- to help the body move freely.

For these three independent functions, the skeleton, muscles and nerves are interconnected in a mechanism that is far more complex than even the most sophisticated machine.

SPINAL TRAINING

The aim of Spinal Training is to find the right balance between the two forces mentioned above in order to improve the performance of the back and the entire body (see Chapter 4 for more information and Chapter 6 for exercises in the program). The principles of grounding (linked to gravitational force) and elongation (ground reaction force) are essential.

IN SUMMARY

- Evolution has led us toward increasingly elaborate movements. Our bodies are made for movement and not for remaining seated for hours.
- Inactivity is increasingly the norm in industrialized societies.
- Exercise is the first line of defense against inactivity.

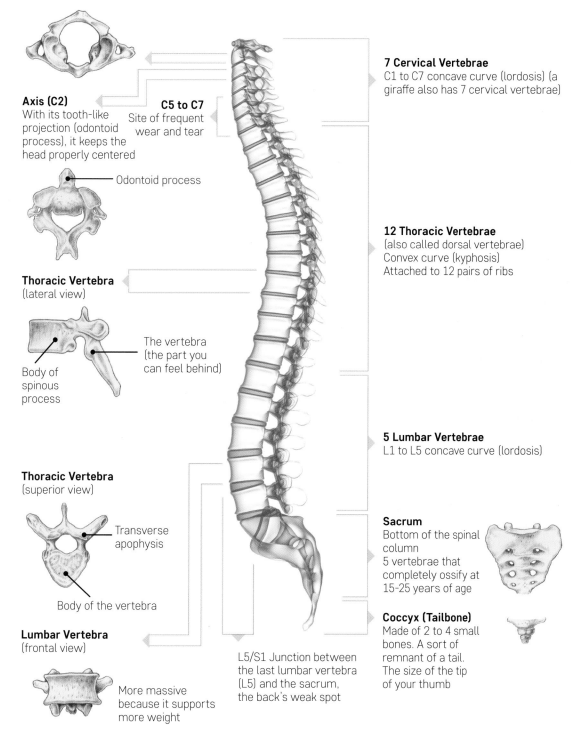

Atlas (C1)
First cervical vertebra
Supports the skull, in the way that
Atlas supported the weight of the Earth
on his shoulders (Greek mythology)

✳
Vertex
Top of the skull

7 Cervical Vertebrae
C1 to C7 concave curve (lordosis) (a
giraffe also has 7 cervical vertebrae)

Axis (C2)
With its tooth-like
projection (odontoid
process), it keeps the
head properly centered

C5 to C7
Site of frequent
wear and tear

Odontoid process

Thoracic Vertebra
(lateral view)

The vertebra
(the part you
can feel behind)

Body of
spinous
process

12 Thoracic Vertebrae
(also called dorsal vertebrae)
Convex curve (kyphosis)
Attached to 12 pairs of ribs

5 Lumbar Vertebrae
L1 to L5 concave curve (lordosis)

Thoracic Vertebra
(superior view)

Transverse
apophysis

Body of the vertebra

Sacrum
Bottom of the spinal
column
5 vertebrae that
completely ossify at
15-25 years of age

Lumbar Vertebra
(frontal view)

More massive
because it supports
more weight

L5/S1 Junction between
the last lumbar vertebra
(L5) and the sacrum,
the back's weak spot

Coccyx (Tailbone)
Made of 2 to 4 small
bones. A sort of
remnant of a tail.
The size of the tip
of your thumb

Back Muscles

The back is well equipped with muscles. Here they are, layer by layer, from the most superficial to the deepest.

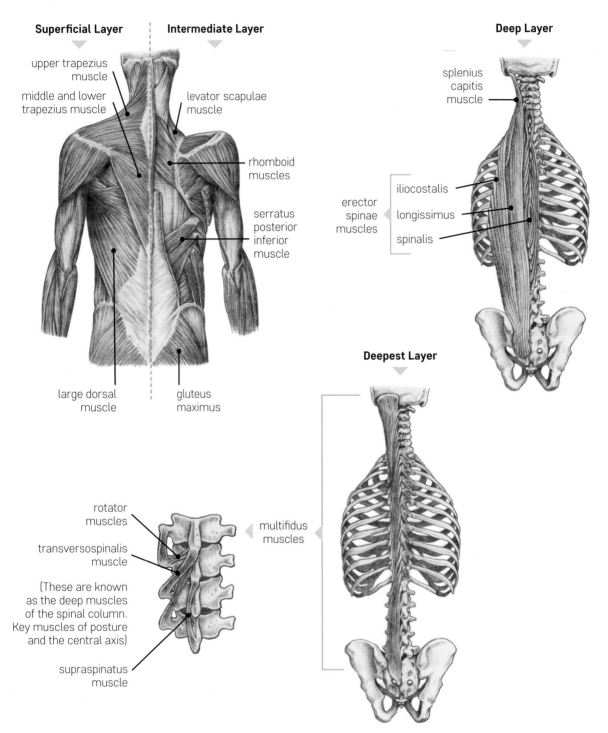

Superficial Layer

Intermediate Layer

upper trapezius muscle

middle and lower trapezius muscle

levator scapulae muscle

rhomboid muscles

serratus posterior inferior muscle

large dorsal muscle

gluteus maximus

Deep Layer

splenius capitis muscle

erector spinae muscles

iliocostalis

longissimus

spinalis

Deepest Layer

rotator muscles

transversospinalis muscle

(These are known as the deep muscles of the spinal column. Key muscles of posture and the central axis)

supraspinatus muscle

multifidus muscles

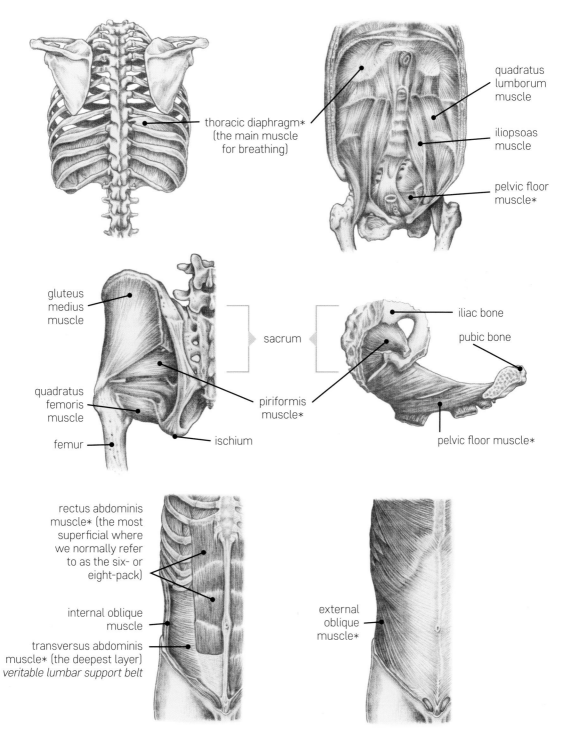

thoracic diaphragm* (the main muscle for breathing)

quadratus lumborum muscle

iliopsoas muscle

pelvic floor muscle*

gluteus medius muscle

quadratus femoris muscle

femur

sacrum

piriformis muscle*

ischium

iliac bone

pubic bone

pelvic floor muscle*

rectus abdominis muscle* (the most superficial where we normally refer to as the six- or eight-pack)

internal oblique muscle

transversus abdominis muscle* (the deepest layer) *veritable lumbar support belt*

external oblique muscle*

* Core muscles (see pages 79–81)

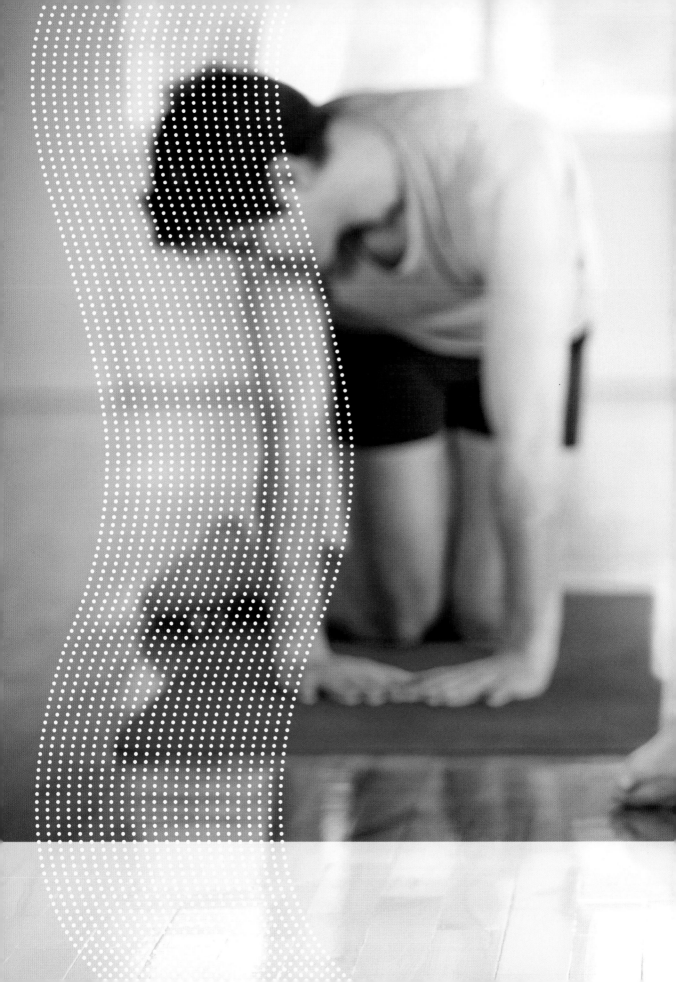

CHAPTER 2: UNDERSTANDING BACK
PROBLEMS TO HELP PREVENT THEM

What Causes Pain?

There are a multitude of reasons for backaches and back conditions, but a Tylenol deficiency isn't one of them! While not every subject covered in this chapter will apply to your situation, it is very unlikely that none of them do (if that's the case, consider yourself lucky!). Just the same, a better understanding of the main causes of backache, however, can help you prevent them.

What Are the Real Causes of Back Problems?

Do you think having weak abdominal muscles explains your backache, or that all problems stem from a blocked vertebra? Not necessarily.

Here, you'll find the 18 principal causes of back pain, divided into five categories: lifestyle; physical (activity or external physical stress); physiological (the body's internal functions); anatomical (skeleton and muscles); and emotional.

> Not all causes will apply to your situation, but it is very unlikely that none of them do.

Lifestyle Causes
- inactivity
- smoking
- excess weight

Physical Causes
- poor posture
- poor execution of movements
- handling heavy loads
- accidents
- vibrations
- a non-ergonomic workplace/ office

Physiological Causes
- organ problems
- hormonal changes
- blocked vertebrae
- poor vision
- adhesions

Anatomical Causes
- a short leg
- scoliosis
- muscle imbalances

Emotional Cause
- stress

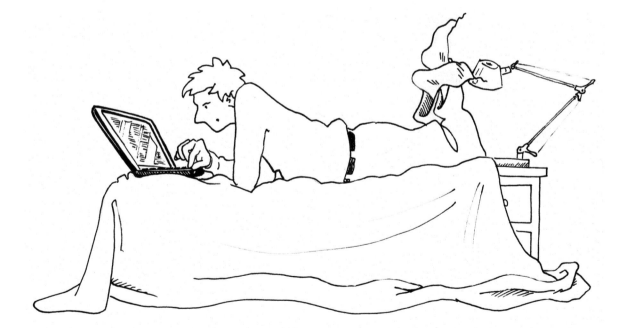

Lifestyle Causes

Inactivity

Inactivity is a curse that is associated with so many health problems (obesity, diabetes, etc.), and it continues to make a significant impact on a worldwide scale. The back, body and mind require a minimum amount of physical activity in order to function properly. In short, to be healthy, you have to move.

Smoking

Everyone knows that smoking is linked to lung disease (including cancer), but did you know that tobacco is also one of the back's greatest enemies? The many chemicals and toxic substances in cigarettes do more than affect the lungs in a harmful way — they also put stress on the entire body. Two studies have shown that heavy smokers have a spinal column and organs that are less mobile.

Excess Weight

Excess weight is principally linked to lifestyle, even when other factors (such as genetics) are determined as partly responsible. Along with its negative impact on the mechanics of the back, excess weight puts additional strain on the entire body, especially the heart. Body fat requires its share of blood and nutrients. Carrying an extra 44 pounds (20 kg) is therefore more demanding on the body than just carrying a knapsack of the same weight. It's a well-known fact that obesity greatly increases the risk of cardiovascular problems and diabetes, but what is less known is that obesity is also a predisposing factor in osteoarthritis, due to the heavy load placed on the joints. The knees, pelvis and back are particularly affected. If that weren't enough, obesity is also associated with an increase in tissue inflammation, which can cause back problems. In North America, about 60% of individuals carry excess weight, spiking the risk of health problems, and the proportion of obese people has more than doubled in 20 years. Even though the statistics are less disastrous in Europe and the rest of the world, the changes that have been observed in those regions' eating habits and a lifestyle that is increasingly sedentary are charting steady gains in obesity.

Therapeutic Advice

As a physical therapist, I've seen how back exercises don't always work for heavy smokers. If you smoke, consider quitting as soon as possible. Cigarettes put a lot of stress on the entire body.

Spinal Training Tip

After quitting smoking, the body goes through withdrawal and needs time to detoxify and rebalance. This can last from a few weeks to a full year, depending on the individual. During this period, certain exercises help get the body back on an even keel. Spinal Training addresses these, with an emphasis on breathing and mobility exercises, without forgetting about cardio. However, they need to be slowly incorporated into a routine, since the withdrawal symptoms may increase during this period of readjustment.

Physical Therapist's View

One of my patients, a very talented professional dancer, had the habit of smoking while on tour, and quitting a few days after returning home. There would be several cycles during the year. I could tell by examining him if he was in a smoking or non-smoking phase, not by smell but by the mobility of his vertebrae. His upper dorsal vertebrae were always tense when he was smoking, and they went back to moving freely a few days after he quit. Luckily, he has since stopped smoking, but during all those years his spinal column never lied to me.

Physical Causes

Poor Posture

It's rare to see someone today with good posture. With our current lifestyle, poor posture is one of the principal causes of backache. What is good posture and how can we save our back from a long and slow deterioration? Posture is so important that I've devoted an entire chapter on it (see Chapter 3).

Poor Execution of Movements

It can take just one movement, such as yanking a tire out of the trunk of your car, to injure your back. Even something as innocuous as picking up a pencil from the floor can trigger intense back pain. In either case, you should consider the probability of an underlying cause. The familiar movement when your back suddenly "locks up" is often the proverbial straw that broke the camel's back.

Repetitive movements are even more often at fault. Think of the time you resumed playing a sport again, such as tennis, or the day you spent 12 hours gardening. As a general rule, a well-trained body that executes a movement in the right way, even many times over, does not get injured. Think of pro tennis star Roger Federer and the amazing fluidity of each of his gestures. It is not surprising that he is one of the only professional players who has sustained very few injuries in decades of play.

Therapeutic Advice

Consult your doctor or kinesiologist to get an accurate assessment of your excess weight. A combination of exercise and changes in your eating habits (we're not talking about dieting here) is the best solution.

Spinal Training Tip

Cardiovascular training is the basis of all weight-loss programs. Combining it with muscle-strengthening exercises improves your chances of success.

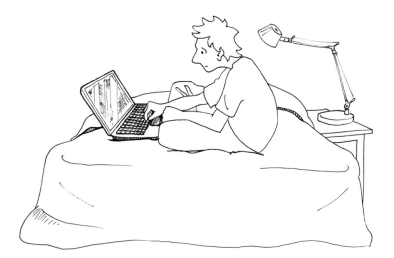

Spinal Training Tip

The principles of Spinal Training can be applied to all your movements, and help you execute them with fluidity and control, while protecting your back. Strengthen and activate the body's core muscles as well as the deep muscles of the spinal column.

Handling Heavy Loads

The heavier the load you lift, the greater the risk to your back, especially if the load is held away from the body. Supporting a load far from the body increases the load placed on the extended arms and multiplies the strain on the back tenfold. The intervertebral disks, which act as shock absorbers in between vertabrae, in particular, can be damaged, causing further problems. Imagine yourself placing an enormous turkey in the oven, holding the pan with your arms fully extended. Just the thought of it can cause your back to seize up! If you think having powerful biceps will protect you, you should know that they will only come in handy for holding the load, but they won't prevent your back from straining.

The principles of handling loads:

- The load remains as close to the body as possible;
- The body has a stable base thanks to the feet, which are firmly planted on the floor (see page 57);
- The spinal column always stays within the "base" area formed by the feet. It must not extend past that area.
- The back is straight at all times, with the spinal column elongated (see page 60);
- The core muscles are activated (see page 79).

Therapeutic Advice

How to handle a load while keeping the legs and center of the body anchored.

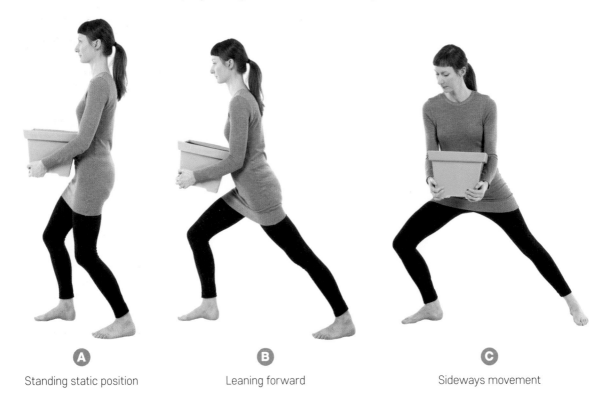

A	B	C
Standing static position	Leaning forward	Sideways movement

Accidents

Not surprising, an accident can cause temporary or permanent damage to your back. It's rare that you'll slip through life unscathed — recall the time you were in a fender bender, or the time you foolishly bounced down the stairs on your rear end.

It was over so quickly, but did it ever hurt! Sometimes, back pain creeps up on you weeks or months after an accident. Let's take the classic example of a car accident when someone is hit from behind, causing whiplash. Once the stiffness has passed, usually one to four weeks later, a more serious problem is likely to set in. The body decides to send an alarm signal — pain — to alert you that it is no longer capable of compensating for this situation that has occurred some time ago. For example, if the accident has left you with a misaligned pelvis, blocked vertebrae and a tense diaphragm, you may be able to endure it for awhile, but your body ultimately has its limits in its ability to adapt.

Vibrations

Being exposed to vibrations from motorized vehicles, airplanes or other machinery poses an even greater risk to the back than sitting for long periods of time. Vibrations can cause long-term damage to the intervertebral disks. Helicopter pilots are on the front line in terms of risk. They are followed by truck drivers and people who drive their car for long hours, the car being one of the principal sources of vibrations in our society. Being stuck in a sitting position, with continuous vibrations, the right foot on alert on the pedal and the stress of driving is a potent cocktail for back tension. Have you previously experienced tension in your neck or lower back or felt the familiar sharp pain in your buttocks on a two-hour car trip? If you have, you should know that these are very common symptoms.

A Non-Ergonomic Workplace

Ergonomy is the science that studies the relationship between humans, their work methods and their work environment. Having an ergonomic workplace is essential for the back. It should allow us to perform our tasks in comfort while being efficient in our movements. You may have the most physically fit back in the world and the most fluid movements, but if your workplace is not adapted to your posture and the way you move, it can lead to back problems in the long term. A number of studies have shown the causal relationship between back problems and working in a sitting or standing position. A poorly laid-out workstation (which is a frequent issue), a work surface that is too low (as in the case of a cook), or materials/packages that require one to lift them too far away from the body can all be very harmful to the back. It can be useful to consult an ergonomist to make the proper adjustments to your work space.

Therapeutic Advice

After a serious accident, even if the symptoms disappear, see a physical therapist, who will ensure there are no physical aftereffects.

Spinal Training Tip

Avoid vigorous exercise after an accident. Give your body a chance to heal. Relax with balancing or breathing exercises.

Therapeutic Advice

If you are exposed to intense and frequent vibrations, such as in the case of a truck driver, make sure you have an adapted seat like a pneumatic one, which diminishes the impact of the vibrations.

Spinal Training Tip

Exercises to elongate the spinal column and stretching exercises are highly recommended, along with strengthening the core muscles and deep muscles of the spinal column. See Routine K on page 233 for exercises that are easy to do while driving.

Spinal Training Tip

On page 234, you'll find the Q routine, featuring many exercises that can be done during work hours. These mini-breaks will help you maintain your energy, keep your muscles relaxed and care for your back.

Physiological Causes

Organ Problems

A backache can be linked to a problem in an organ in three ways. First, a sick organ can make the back, abdomen, chest or pelvis hurt in an area that is usually similar in every individual. This is called referred pain. At the same time, if you have pain in one spot, that does not necessarily mean that the corresponding organ is sick. The origin of the referred pain lies mainly in an imbalance in the nervous system linked to the abnormal function of an organ. We are not talking about pathology, but rather physiology (body function).

Secondly, each organ is linked through nerves to an area in the spinal column. Chronic irritation in an organ can cause a change in the nerve signal in the corresponding area of the spinal column. Let's take the example of the stomach. The nerves in this organ originate in vertebrae situated between your scapulae, or shoulder blades, (vertebrae T5 to T9, to be precise) and the base of your skull. A chronic gastric reflux problem can cause some people pain between the scapulae (particularly on the left side). It is interesting to note that the inverse relation also exists. Therefore, a vertebral blockage between the scapulae can eventually lead to a problem with stomach function.

Thirdly, an organ problem can have mechanical repercussions on the back. Organs are not suspended as if by magic in our body. They are actually all directly or indirectly attached to the spinal column, chest, pelvis or skull. Tension in an organ can produce mechanical tension in the back. For example, someone who has pneumonia may have pain in the chest and in the dorsal vertebrae (the lungs are directly under the ribs). Fragile intestines, with significant bloating, can cause tension in the lower back (the intestines are attached to the lower back). Finally, tension in the esophagus can cause tension between the scapulae.

Points of Referred Pain

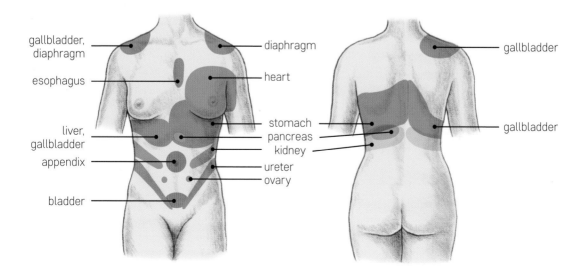

Examples of links between the organs and the spinal column.

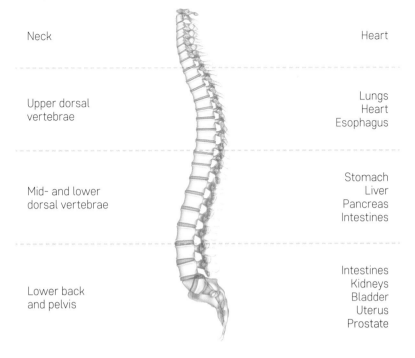

Spinal Column	Organs
Neck	Heart
Upper dorsal vertebrae	Lungs / Heart / Esophagus
Mid- and lower dorsal vertebrae	Stomach / Liver / Pancreas / Intestines
Lower back and pelvis	Intestines / Kidneys / Bladder / Uterus / Prostate

Spinal Training Tip

Physical activity, in general, encourages organs, which detest inactivity, to function well. Spinal Training helps organs move more freely and stimulates them to function effectively.

Hormonal Changes

The hormonal system is a complex network in the body. Here is a brief summary of how it works: With the help of its big team players (the hypothalamus, pituitary gland, thyroid, pancreas, adrenal glands, uterus and ovaries or testicles), the hormonal system secretes hormones that regulate growth, development and reproduction. To maintain the body's equilibrium, it works in conjunction with the nervous system and immune system. In the case of hormonal changes, a host of symptoms can be observed, including tension or pain in the back.

A few examples of possible links with the back:

- premenstrual syndrome: back and pelvic pain
- premenopause and menopause: muscle stiffness or back pain
- adolescence: muscle stiffness or back pain

Blocked Vertebrae

As you've read until now, and contrary to popular belief, not all back pain is linked to vertebral blockage. Nevertheless, backaches can occur from a blockage between two or more vertebrae, at the level of the ribs, the pelvis (sacroiliac joints and pubic bone) or the sternum. In fact, we can find blockages in all the joints in the body, from the ears to the jaw, and from the knees to the hips. All these blockages hinder movement in the body and have an indirect impact on the back.

Therapeutic Advice

Consult your doctor for a checkup to ensure your hormonal levels are functioning normally.

Spinal Training Tip

Physical activity regulates the secretion of a number of hormones. To help balance the hormonal system, the emphasis should be on exercises for neuromuscular relaxation, flexibility and mobility, as well as cardiovascular exercises.

Therapeutic Advice

Consult a physical therapist to have a precise evaluation of your back. Remember that the long-term objective is not to depend on the therapist to take care of your spinal column.

Spinal Training Tip

Spinal Training is excellent for preventing vertebral blockages. Mobility, posture and spinal column elongation exercises are the key.

Therapeutic Advice

See an optometrist/ ophthalmologist for an eye examination. If you have progressive lenses, discuss the possibility of getting reading glasses just for working at the computer, as well as any other required glasses for everyday use.

Spinal Training Tip

Exercises to relax the muscles of the neck, skull and face are recommended.

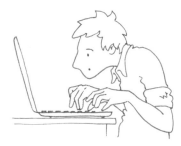

Here, the head is projected forward to compensate for poor vision.

The blockage itself can have several causes: incorrect movement, poor posture, accident, muscle imbalance, organ problem, etc. Do these problems sound familiar? You may think that the blockage is the result of a more serious problem, and that may be the case, but once the cause of the blockage is resolved, the blockage itself may remain and continue to cause pain. What's more, the pain will not necessarily be felt in the exact spot as the blockage. It may be located in the area that is compensating for the blockage.

Compensation is the body's reaction to a problem that helps the body maintain its normal position and movements. For example, a pain between the scapulae can result in compensation for a blockage located higher up (at the base of the neck, for example), or lower down (in the lumbar vertebrae, for example). A pain in one sacroiliac joint (in the pelvis) can result in a blockage in the other sacroiliac joint. We are often fooled as to where the pain originates.

As an osteopath, I treat these sorts of problems every day. The majority of people who come to me regarding a back problem have a least one vertebral blockage in the initial evaluation, and that the location of their pain rarely indicates the origin of the problem.

Poor Vision

Posture and back comfort can be affected by poor vision or by improperly adjusted eyeglasses or contact lenses. The most common example is working at a computer. Surely, there have been times when you've found yourself, after spending a few hours in front of the computer, with your head projecting forward and your spine curved because your eyes are tired. If your vision is affected, this poor posture can worsen and become almost permanent, which is not good news for your back. Presbyopia — the loss of ability by the eyes' lens to focus sharply on nearby objects, particularly in middle age — is particularly problematic. The resulting tensions can be found throughout the back, and especially at the base of the skull. In addition, progressive lenses make the eyes and neck work in a way that does not respect the body's natural movements. The eyes do not move naturally, which causes more tension in the neck and even in the muscles of the skull and face.

Adhesions

An adhesion is an area where layers of tissues that are normally separate are stuck together due to inflammation, preventing them from easily sliding against each other. The body tries involuntarily to "close up" the area with an adhesion. This creates an imbalance in posture, which affects the back. In the case of an adhesion on the right side of the abdomen, for example, an appendicitis scar, it is likely that the person has "closed up" over the scar on his right side. He must really work to strengthen all his back muscles to stand up straight, and if the adhesion remains, his posture will always be affected. There are two types of adhesions: scars and internal adhesion.

Scars

Not all scars are adherent, but when there is significant inflammation associated with scarring, they can become adherent. If you have a scar (cesarean, appendectomy, gallbladder removed, epidural, liposuction, breast implants, a facelift, cut, etc.), you can test yourself to see if it is adherent.

Internal Adhesions

The same phenomenon of tissues sticking together can occur without any exterior incision. Here, chronic internal inflammation is often the cause and can affect a variety of areas. For example, an adhesion in the large intestine can result in an inflammatory disease (Crohn's disease or celiac disease). Adhesions of the pleura (coating of the lung), the lungs and the chest can occur after pneumonia or chronic bronchitis, and frequent urinary tract infections can cause adhesions in the area of the bladder and pubic bone. Many people don't even know they have internal adhesions. They can lead to repercussions on the back, because as we've seen, any adhesion can modify posture and body movement.

Anatomical Causes

A Short Leg

If you have your pant legs hemmed at two different lengths or if you have scoliosis (see the next page), you may have a short leg. It is estimated that 4 to 12% of people have one leg shorter or longer (depending on your point of view) than the other. This condition is also known as "leg length inequality" (LLI). This inequality causes an imbalance in the posture, which forces the body to work harder to compensate in order to stand upright. This situation does not necessarily cause back pain, but the greater the difference between the two legs, the greater the risk of eventually developing a back problem.

Therapeutic Advice

To learn whether you have one or more adhesions, consult a therapist who has been trained to evaluate and treat this problem, such as an osteopath, a physiotherapist or a kinesitherapist.

Spinal Training Tip

External scar adhesions are easy enough to work on without the guidance of a physical therapist. You only need to pinch the skin and roll it between your fingers for about 30 seconds daily. Focus on the areas that are the most "stuck." Keep pinching and rolling every day, until the skin regains the normal suppleness of the surrounding skin. It is best to leave internal adhesions to the care of a physical therapist.

Therapeutic Advice

If you think you have a short leg, a physical therapist (osteopath, physiotherapist, kinesitherapist, chiropractor) can evaluate you and a doctor can order a scan of the lower limbs (measuring the bones from an X-ray) to have a more precise idea of the difference. If the difference is more than three-quarters of an inch (2 cm), it is suggested that you consult an orthotist for a corrective orthotic device.

Spinal Training Tip

Balance exercises using one leg at a time are recommended, in order to rebalance the body in relation to each leg (see page 192).

Therapeutic Advice

A physical therapist (osteopath, physiotherapist, kinesitherapist, chiropractor) can determine if you have scoliosis and the type of scoliosis. It's a good idea to see your doctor and ask for an X-ray to determine the exact angle of the scoliosis.

Spinal Training Tip

Spinal Training can assist in correcting or slowing down the progress of scoliosis. It helps to rebalance the muscles in the back, restore movement to the vertebrae and elongate the spinal column.

A difference of about three-quarters of an inch (2 cm) can affect posture in a significant way. Starting at 2 inches (5 cm) of difference, the problem is considered to be severe. Some studies suggest that even a difference of about a quarter to half an inch (0.5 to 1 cm) is enough to increase the incidence of back problems.

A short leg is often the result of a fracture in a lower limb before or during the growth period. Depending on the area of the fracture (tibia, fibula or femur), the healed bone may remain shorter in the limb than the corresponding bone of the other limb. A short leg can also be caused by long-term poor posture or intense practice of an asymmetrical sport (tennis, fencing, high-jump, etc).

Scoliosis

Scoliosis is a visible, S-shaped curve in the spine. It is most frequently found in women and often develops during adolescence. When it is severe, it can require surgery (inserting rods along the spinal column) or a corrective brace to be worn for a long period of time. Scoliosis is sometimes associated with a short leg, but just like having a short leg, it does not necessarily cause back pain. The more severe it is, however, the greater the risk of pain, as the body must compensate for the curvature and back movements are limited. There are two types of scoliosis: structural (real) scoliosis is caused by a deformity in the vertebrae. Habit scoliosis is due to imbalance in the deep muscles of the spinal column and can be corrected by exercise.

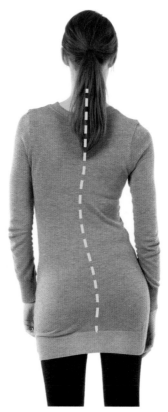

Scoliosis due to a short leg

Muscle Imbalances

We often hear that a back problem is due to weak muscles, which is sometimes true. More important than muscle strength or endurance, however, is muscle balance, which is essential in helping the back function properly. To put it another way, it is better to have average and equal strength on both sides of the body than a lot of strength on the right side and just average strength on the left side. Ultimately, we seek balance in the body over three dimensions. This balance is associated with good posture.

If you move asymmetrically in a repetitive fashion, such as in racquet sports, throwing, archery, etc., this can lead to muscle imbalance over time. Studies have shown the difference in bone length and muscle volume between the two arms of tennis players. The research has prompted trainers to design muscle-building programs for athletes that help rebalance their muscles. The same can be seen in people who habitually sit with their weight on one buttock and always cross the same leg over the other. In doing so, they risk causing muscle imbalance in the pelvis and back over time.

Therapeutic Advice

Practicing a sport will always have more positive than negative effects. Continue to play the sports you love and rebalance your body with Spinal Training. Strengthen and activate your core muscles as well as the deep muscles of your spinal column, and maintain good posture.

Emotional Cause

Stress

Stress has a direct impact on every part of the body, including the back. Faced with stress, the body's regulatory systems mobilize: the hormonal system sets off a chain reaction and the alerted nervous system goes into sympathetic mode (with the familiar surge of adrenaline). The phenomenon is known as the fight-or-flight reaction.

This response to stress helped our species hunt prehistoric beasts — and to run way from them. It is a reaction linked to the survival instinct, which is deeply embedded in our entire being. The problem is, when faced with emotional stress, our nervous and hormonal systems react in the same way, as though they were facing a life-threatening situation. But instead of fighting or taking flight to expend this stored-up energy, we often remain quite passive and muscles, especially deep muscles, tense up. This creates tension in the back that can cause discomfort or pain. The increased tension in the deep muscles can also cause one or more blockages between the vertebrae, preventing them from moving freely. Blockages can also be found in the chest (one blocked side is especially painful) or the pelvis.

Spinal Training Tip

An important role of physical activity is to release stress. Put the emphasis on cardio, balance and breathing exercises — and have fun!

If stress is repetitive, the problem can become chronic and affect other areas of the body. The spinal column houses the spinal cord, which is inseparable from the nervous system, so it can have a number of consequences for the back and beyond. In a chronic situation, one or more areas become rigid and almost immobile. The back thus loses its ability to move, the muscles tense up and other problems, such as digestive problems, fatigue, memory loss, weight gain and an increase in blood pressure, can develop.

Tension or blockages are often produced in the same areas in the body. They are considered a person's fragile zones or weak spots. People who live through similar emotional stress, however, can react differently. For example, in the case of intense stress at work combined with a high risk of losing a job, one person may wake up one morning with a torticollis, or stiff neck. Another will feel a familiar sharp pain between her shoulder blades on the right side (her fragile zone being the mid-dorsal muscles). Someone else might have stiffness in his lower back that prevents him from doing normal activities (his fragile zone is in the lumbar muscles). And yet another may have no tension in the back at all. Each person/body handles stress differently.

Other Causes

The following elements should also be mentioned as potentially problematic for the back:

- wearing an orthotic device that isn't properly fitting;
- wearing inappropriate shoes;
- carrying heavy or awkward bags;
- infections or illnesses;
- congenital malformations.

IN SUMMARY

Backache is not due to one cause, nor is there one solution for it. What brings on pain and how to treat it successfully will vary from person to person, in part because of the complexity of the relationships between the body's different systems. If you have back pain, seek the help of a specialized health professional who can evaluate your condition and treat it accordingly. The goal in these cases is to help you regain control of your health without becoming dependent on a physical therapist. Just the same, sometimes you need a helping hand — the information in this chapter and exercises illustrated later in the book will get you on the road to recovery.

If you lead an active life, if you manage stress well, if you take the time to relax and you walk, dance and maintain good posture, then you very likely already have most of the solution within your reach. The strains of our current lifestyle, however, demand more, and it is becoming increasingly important to do an exercise routine for the back regularly in order to keep it healthy.

When Should You See A Doctor For Your Back?

Although treating back pain as soon as possible can offer some relief, identifying the cause of your back problem is also important. Your family doctor can make a diagnosis, recommend treatment (medication, surgery, physical therapy, etc.), order tests if necessary (X-ray, CT-scan, MRI, etc.) or refer you to a specialist (orthopedist, neurologist, etc.). Most of all, your doctor should rule out any serious condition underlying your back pain. You should immediately see a doctor if your back pain is associated with one of the following:

- fever;
- pain following an accident;
- headaches;
- pain following a blow to the head;
- unexplained weight loss;
- weakness, numbness or tingling in a leg or arm;
- urinary incontinence;
- loss of sensation in a limb;
- increased sensitivity when touching an area in the spinal column;
- pain that intensifies during the night.

The Categories of Pain

Acute pain (lasts up to 4 weeks)	Subacute pain* (lasts from 4 weeks to 3 months)	Chronic pain (persists more than 3 months)
The term "acute" should not be confused with the intensity of the pain. About 90% of pains disappear in 4 weeks or less.	More or less constant pain that, in some cases, develops into chronic pain.	Constant pain that lasts more than 3 months. Five to 10% of cases become chronic.

* The term "subacute pain" is often grouped with acute pain. This choice of terminology has been used in this book in order to simplify the text. Hereafter, we refer to acute or chronic pain.

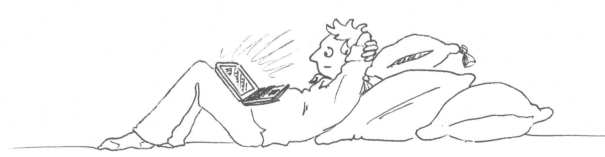

Possible Diagnoses

Whether the cause of the pain is known or not, it is much easier to come up with a plan of action once a diagnosis has been made. A better understanding of the diagnoses related to your back problem will help you choose the most appropriate exercises and avoid certain potentially harmful movements.

Lumbago, Dorsalgia Or Cervicalgia

The suffix "algia" comes from the Greek *algos* and means "pain." Lumbago is a pain in the lumbar region (lower back). Dorsalgia is a pain in the dorsal or chest region, and cervicalgia means neck pain. Any of these diagnoses take into account only the presence of pain, without enlightening us as to their origin.

Sciatic Neuralgia

Also called sciatica or sciatic neuritis, sciatic neuralgia is pain along the sciatic nerve. The pain most often radiates from the lower back, hip, buttocks and down the leg. It can travel down to the toes and even cause intense pain in the buttocks and lower back. Sciatic neuralgia most often shows up in just one leg, usually on the side where the sciatic nerve is irritated. The irritation generally originates in the lower back, in the area of the last lumbar vertebrae and the sacrum. It can also be due to tension in the deep gluteal muscles, particularly in the area of the piriformis muscle. (The sciatic nerve passes just under the piriformis muscle and, in some individuals, through the muscle.)

The symptoms manifest themselves most often as throbbing pain, numbness or weakness in the lower limb that is affected. It can be exacerbated by coughing, sneezing, handling heavy loads or poor posture.

Spinal Training Tip

Focus on exercises that elongate the spinal column. Mobility and breathing exercises are also recommended. Certain flexibility exercises are particularly effective.

Lumbar Sprain (Dorsal or Cervical)

A sprain occurs when one or more ligaments are stretched or torn. Think of an ankle sprain, but it occurring in the back. A lumbar sprain generally occurs after making an awkward twisting movement while supporting a heavy load. Note that this diagnosis is often made in a general way for pain in the lower back even though there may not be any ligament damage. A cervical sprain is most often caused by a car accident — with impact from the front or the back — and is referred to as "whiplash."

Spinal Training Tip

In case of a sprain, avoid stretching the injured area, since stretching a ligament that has already been stretched or torn can aggravate the injury. Emphasis should be placed on gentle mobility exercises along with breathing and posture exercises.

Herniated Disk

A herniated disk occurs when the gelatinous core of the disk forces its way through the fibers of the annulus fibrosus to project outward from the disk.

Spinal Training Tip

In the case of a herniated disk, "sit-up" abdominal strengthening exercises and certain other muscle strengthening exercises should be avoided. Some gentle stretching is recommended, but it should not increase the pain at any time. Elongation exercises are also recommended.

The hernia does not necessarily cause pain, but if it contains a nerve, it can cause pain in the sensitive area of the nerve. The area by far most often affected by herniated disks is the lower back. A herniated disk at this level normally causes pain on the side and behind the leg and can lead to sciatic neuralgia.

Symptoms associated with a herniated disk include numbness, tingling or muscle weakness. Hernias are also frequent in the cervical vertebrae, but much less frequent in the dorsal vertebrae. In the case of a cervical hernia, the pain is often felt in an arm. Pain is more common on one side only, particularly on the side where the nerve is irritated.

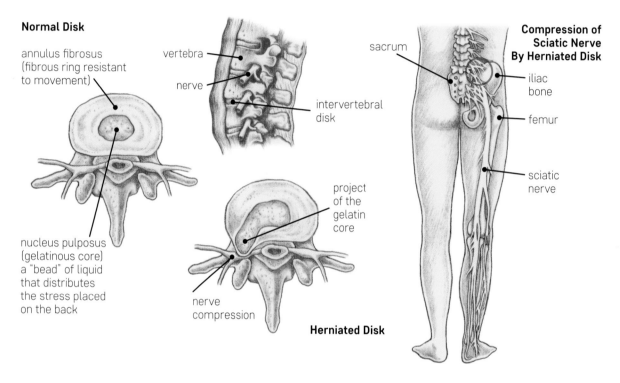

Normal Disk

annulus fibrosus (fibrous ring resistant to movement)

nucleus pulposus (gelatinous core) a "bead" of liquid that distributes the stress placed on the back

vertebra

nerve

intervertebral disk

project of the gelatin core

nerve compression

Herniated Disk

sacrum

Compression of Sciatic Nerve By Herniated Disk

iliac bone

femur

sciatic nerve

Arthritis

Spinal Training Tip

Spinal Training is suitable in cases of arthritis. Emphasize exercises for breathing, flexibility, mobility and posture. In the case of acute pain, follow the routines designed for relief (D3, L3, N3) (see page 209).

The word "arthritis" comes from the Greek word *arthron*, which means "joint," and itis, which means "inflammatory ailment." Arthritis is an inflammatory ailment that can take a variety of forms. The two most common forms are osteoarthritis (wearing down type) and rheumatoid polyarthritis (inflammatory type). A form of arthritis called ankylosing spondylitis, also known as bamboo spine, particularly affects the back. With this condition, the spinal column bends and the vertebrae end up fusing together, producing a severely curved spine.

The first person known to have suffered from ankylosing spondylitis was Ramses II. Radiological exams made by a Belgian team showed that, in 1236 BC, the pharaoh's spinal column had to be fractured when his body was being embalmed, because his spinal column was curved and fused.

Osteoarthritis

Osteoarthritis is a condition that affects the joints and leads to loss of mobility. If there is inflammation, it can also cause pain. Osteoarthritis is a degenerative, wearing-down form of arthritis. The cartilage, which prevents the bones from rubbing together, and the bones themselves wear down due to a number of factors. Osteoarthritis is often seen in the neck and the lower back. It can also affect other joints, including the hips and knees.

Factors that predispose an individual to osteoarthritis:

- excess weight;
- poor execution of movements;
- poor posture;
- smoking;
- heredity.

Section of spinal column with osteoarthritis

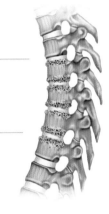

Spinal Training Tip

Spinal Training is suitable in cases of osteoarthritis. Emphasize mobility, flexibility and posture exercises. Cardiovascular training is also essential for controlling weight. Strengthening exercises should be done with a gradual increase in intensity.

Osteoporosis

Osteoporosis is a disease in which the bones become demineralized and fragile. The vertebrae may be affected, which has a direct impact on the back. The bones of the spinal column are most often affected, followed by those of the hips and wrists.

In its early stages, osteoporosis is typically not associated with any symptoms. Fractures are among the biggest concern (often associated with a fall), which affect 40% of women 50 years of age and over. The consequences of the fractures (of the hip, among others) are particularly serious in the elderly.

Bone density tends to decrease by 1 to 2% a year starting at the age of 40. The reduction is more dramatic in women. Following this age, there is a progressive collapsing of the vertebrae, which partly explains why people shrink in height as they age (poor posture and the collapsing of the disks also contribute to this phenomenon).

Spinal Training Tip

Spinal Training is very suitable for osteoporosis. The emphasis is on movements that focus on those areas that are most subjected to gravity because these are the exercises that help increase bone density. They stimulate bone development much more than movements performed in low-gravity situations like water. Walking, running and exercises for posture and strengthening that are done while standing are recommended.

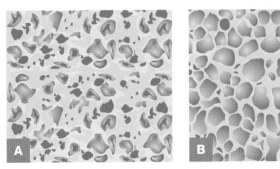

Figure A: Normal bone
Figure B: Demineralized bone (osteoporosis)

Fracture

A major impact to the head, pelvis, back or even the feet can make a vertebra give way, causing a fracture. This serious injury calls for rest and sometimes immobilization, giving the bone a chance to repair itself. In the case of a major injury, in which the bone is severely damaged or if there is nerve compression, surgery may be needed. In more severe cases, an impact can lead to a severe compression of the spinal cord that causes paralysis. You have no doubt heard of people who became paraplegic following a dive into the swimming pool. Unfortunately, it is sometimes only at these moments that we become aware of the importance of the spinal column.

Balancing and breathing exercises are particularly recommended during the consolidation (healing) period of the fracture. Muscle strengthening should be avoided.

Spinal Training Tip

Emphasize exercises to elongate the spinal column. Activating the core muscles also helps protect the injured area. Certain strengthening exercises should be avoided.

Spondylolysis

Coming from the Greek word *spondylos*, which means "vertebra," spondylolysis is a condition in which one vertebra slides over the other. The vertebra most often slides forward, producing stress in the muscles and the disks. The more pronounced the sliding, the greater the risk of pain in the back. When the condition is more severe it is called spondylolysthesis.

Factors that predispose an individual to spondylolysis:

- an accident;
- poor posture;
- handling heavy loads;
- poor execution of movements.

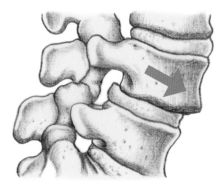

Spondylolysis in a lumbar vertebra

Spinal Training Tip

Stretching the neck muscles during a period of acute torticollis should be avoided. Emphasize exercises that relax the neck, as well as mobility and breathing exercises. Once the acute stage has passed, flexibility and strengthening exercises can be added to the routine.

Torticollis

Torticollis is a condition in which involuntary tension in the neck muscles maintain the neck in an uncomfortable and sometimes twisted position. The muscle most affected is the sternocleidomastoid (SCM). In addition to being an excellent word to toss into a conversation, the SCM greatly limits mobility in the neck when it is tensed. It tilts the head toward the tensed side and twists it to the other side, producing the familiar torticollis posture.

Torticollis in a baby can cause serious posture problems if not treated effectively.

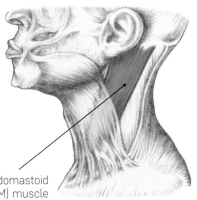

the sternocleidomastoid (SCM) muscle

Explicable Pain

The phenomenon of pain, no matter what the cause (even emotional), can be summed up this way: Pain comes from a change in condition in the body (damaged muscle or ligament, inflammation, infection, etc.). Receptors detect this change and transmit the information through sensory nerves to the areas of the brain responsible for analyzing pain. The brain then orders adjustments to compensate for this pain. This is why an individual unconsciously "closes up" over a painful spot. It is the brain's instinctive attempt to protect this area. The brain's interpretation of the pain can vary according to the person's condition. For example, people who tend to have a negative attitude are more at risk of developing chronic pain.

Spinal Training Tip

The nervous system, including the brain, always intervenes in the pain phenomenon. One of the objectives of Spinal Training is to rebalance the nervous system.

Unexplained Pain

Almost 90% of back pain cannot be seen physically even following the typical lineup of tests (X-ray, CT-scan, MRI, etc.). If you go see your doctor and, after undergoing several tests, he tells you that nothing can explain your problem, you are in the majority. An X-ray will only reveal a problem if there is a visible deformity in the bone. On the other hand, even if you have a spinal column with a normal structure and no sign of wear and tear, that does not guarantee that your spine is moving and functioning well.

IN SUMMARY

- Different types of exercises are recommended depending on the type of injury (diagnosis) and the type of pain (acute or chronic).
- A consultation with a doctor helps to determine the nature of the problem and form a plan of action.

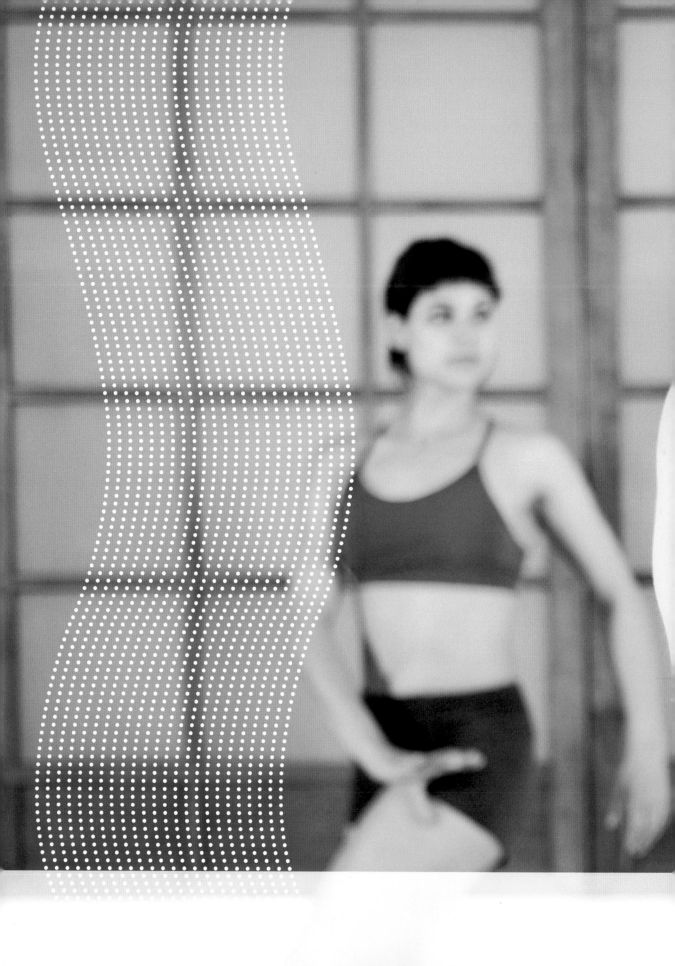

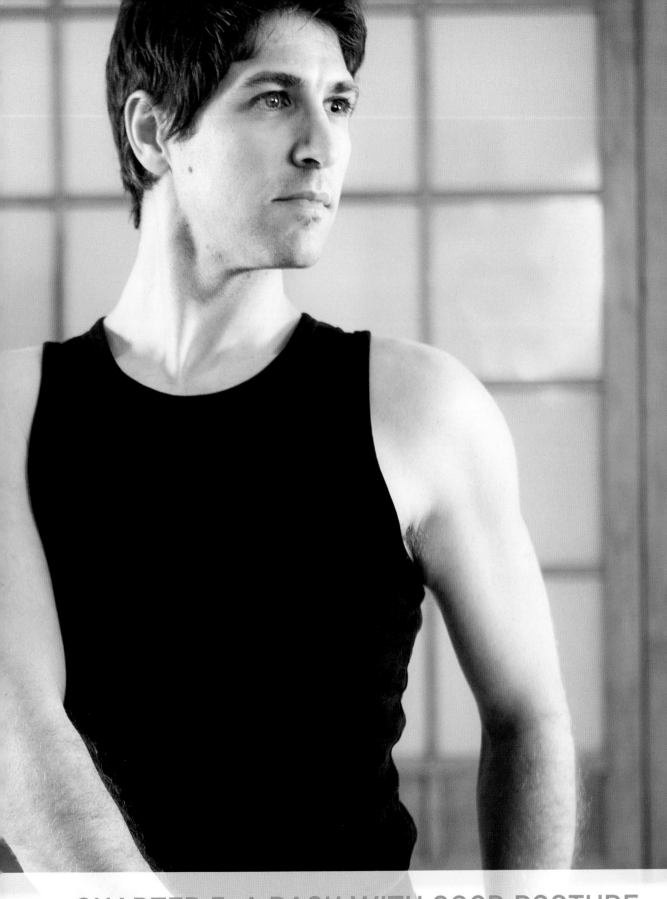

CHAPTER 3: A BACK WITH GOOD POSTURE

From Head
to Toe

Good posture does more for your back and
health, in general, than any "miraculous"
exercise. It's much better to work on improving
your posture (even slightly) than it is to
put yourself through a military regimen of
daily sit-ups in the hopes of developing
strong abdominals.

What Is Posture?

Posture is the position adopted by the body in space. It is most often standing or seated, but can also refer to a multitude of positions taken by the body.

Our posture is our personal signature. You have probably recognized a friend in the distance just by the way she stands. Posture says a lot about personality. Depressive, dynamic, emotional, pliable or entrepreneur — for each temperament there is a posture. Our posture also adapts itself to different events and life situations. The posture we adopt when mourning at a funeral home is different from our posture when making an important presentation in front of an audience, or during a romantic dinner for two.

The effects of good posture include:

- activation of the deep muscles of the back;
- deeper breathing;
- increased efficiency in movements;
- more energy;
- improved digestion;
- greater muscle relaxation;
- improved circulation;
- better appearance.

Examples of Posture

Here are a few examples of posture observed from the side (adapted from the principles of GDS routines — see page 158), with the main muscles activated in the body.

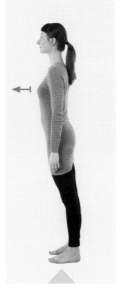

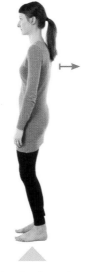

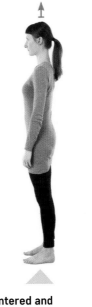

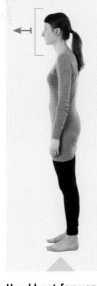

Leaning forward
Tension in the body's posterior muscles

Leaning backward
Tension in the body's anterior muscles

Slumped
General weakening of muscles

Centered and pulled upward
Spinal column straight but barely mobile

Head bent forward
Tension in the neck and chest

Does Your Teenager Slump?

Is your 14-year-old constantly slouching, sporting a curved spine and the silhouette of a sack of potatoes? Does he have the muscle tone of a slug? At the table, does he gobble down tons of food while grunting in an uncivilized manner, but doesn't have the decency to sit up straight? Don't worry. It's all normal. You can blame his hormonal system, which is undergoing profound changes, and one of the effects is atonia (reduced muscle tone). Your teenager has difficulty sitting or standing up straight when he is not stimulated by an activity. Can something be done? It turns out that the best thing for an adolescent during this phase of his life is to do activities that stimulate the body and activate the muscles. It doesn't matter whether it is dancing, tennis, soccer, inline skating or snowboarding, as long as he is moving and it's enjoyable. As for flexibility exercises or yoga, there may not be any added advantages — these activities don't activate the muscles sufficiently and teenagers don't always enjoy the postures.

The Key: Proprioceptors

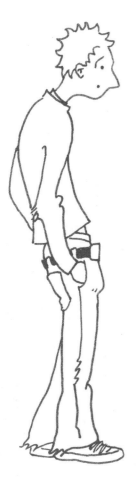

I'm guessing that you've rarely heard of "proprioceptors" but if you only knew how indispensable they were, they might be a regular part of your vocabulary! Proprioceptors are responsible for sensing the changes in your body's position in space and informing the nervous system, which then makes adjustments by commanding the appropriate muscle actions. This process takes place without you even being aware of it and with incredible speed and precision, for example, when your ankle twists and your muscles contract to avoid a sprain (torn ligaments).

Without proprioceptors, which essentially act as sensory receptors, there can be no good posture or coordinated movement. Think of a circus acrobat balancing on one hand, his legs in the air, while he is on top of 20 stacked chairs. His proprioceptors are doing an important job and there's no time for them to take a break.

Proprioceptors are located in key areas of the body. The following diagram shows how certain problems can affect certain principal proprioceptors and destabilize posture. The body must make an extra effort to maintain a stable and balanced position, which puts strain on the back and increases the risk of back problems.

Proprioceptors

When principal proprioceptors are affected with a condition, they can have an impact on posture.

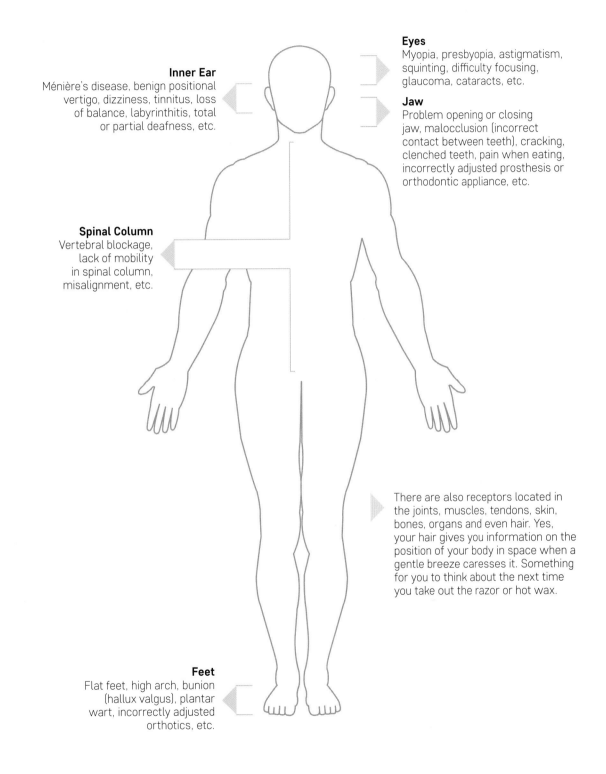

Inner Ear
Ménière's disease, benign positional vertigo, dizziness, tinnitus, loss of balance, labyrinthitis, total or partial deafness, etc.

Eyes
Myopia, presbyopia, astigmatism, squinting, difficulty focusing, glaucoma, cataracts, etc.

Jaw
Problem opening or closing jaw, malocclusion (incorrect contact between teeth), cracking, clenched teeth, pain when eating, incorrectly adjusted prosthesis or orthodontic appliance, etc.

Spinal Column
Vertebral blockage, lack of mobility in spinal column, misalignment, etc.

There are also receptors located in the joints, muscles, tendons, skin, bones, organs and even hair. Yes, your hair gives you information on the position of your body in space when a gentle breeze caresses it. Something for you to think about the next time you take out the razor or hot wax.

Feet
Flat feet, high arch, bunion (hallux valgus), plantar wart, incorrectly adjusted orthotics, etc.

What to remember about proprioceptors:

- Proprioceptors like movement. They need to be stimulated or they will become dormant.
- Proprioceptors work in a team. If one is ineffective, it affects the work of the entire team.
- Properly functioning proprioceptors help you maintain good posture and move more fluidly and efficiently.

Proprioception Training

Spinal Training Tip

Proprioception is an important part of Spinal Training. In this book, for simplicity's sake, no exercise requires equipment. To increase the difficulty of an exercise, you can add a destabilizing accessory (balance disc, BOSU balance trainer, balance ball, etc.).

Training the proprioceptors is called "proprioception," a term that is gradually making its way into general vocabulary. Posture exercises target this aspect.

To train proprioceptors, one has to destabilize at least one member of the team, which forces the other proprioceptors to adapt accordingly. Below is an example of progression in the level of difficulty.

IN SUMMARY

- Each person's posture is his or her personal signature.
- Good posture helps to activate the deep muscles of the back, breathe better and reduce the impact of stress on your spinal column.
- Proprioceptors keep you continuously informed about the position of your body in space.

Proprioception Training

One can increase the work of the proprioceptors in different ways. Here are a few examples, from the easiest to the most difficult.

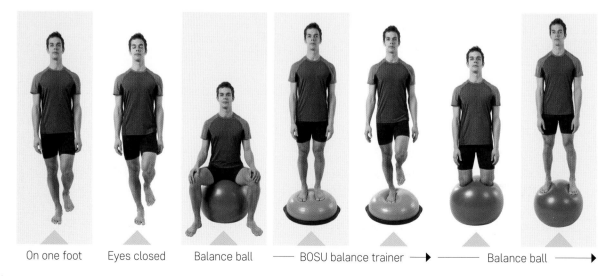

On one foot   Eyes closed   Balance ball   —— BOSU balance trainer ——➤   —— Balance ball ——➤

An Inverted Pendulum

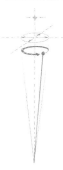

Distinguished kinesiology professor David A. Winter, who was notable for his work in biomedics, studied the control of balance and posture while walking. According to Winter, the body, like a pendulum attached to the ground at the feet, oscillates around this fixed point, with the head representing the mass at the end of a pendulum. He theorized that we oscillate in a cone within a 4-degree vertical angle. The role of the feet is to keep us stable in this cone, and they are able to do this thanks to the information transmitted by the proprioceptors that are found in great number in the soles of the feet and in the joints.

With a slight contraction of the deep muscles of the feet, the pendulum is activated and the body moves as a result. Small changes in the feet cause big changes in posture.

The Neck-Eyes Link

The deep muscles located at the base of the skull (called the suboccipital muscles) are directly linked to eye movements. When one looks to the right, for example, these muscles contract automatically to turn the head to the right. This is known as the oculomotor (or oculocephalogyric) reflex. This phenomenon explains in large part the tensions that accumulate at the base of the skull when the eyes are not properly functioning. The best example of how these muscles affect posture is spending long hours working in front of a computer. The eyes are simply not adapted to looking at a screen for so many hours in a day. The problem intensifies when the screen has not been ergonomically adjusted, which is the case of all laptop computers, or when the screen is not level, too close or too far. In addition to this, many people cannot tolerate looking at a computer screen with progressive lenses. In all cases, unnatural and excessive work for the eyes can lead to tension in the suboccipital muscles, which causes tension at the base of the skull, in the neck and in the head.

Spinal Training Tip

To help your feet, start by not wearing orthotics, but instead training your feet to walk properly and awakening them by mastering the principle of grounding. To do this, an emphasis is placed on proprioception and posture exercises. You also need to adequately stretch the muscles attached to the feet, which have a tendency to be tense. This is followed by muscle reinforcement in a standing position, ensuring that the lower limbs are properly aligned, with the feet solidly planted.

Spinal Training Tip

Certain exercises are very effective for releasing tension associated with the eyes and the base of the skull (see exercises 30, 31 and 32, starting on page 142).

Myth No. 1: Good Floor Exercises = A Good Back

There should not be an emphasis on floor exercises, often in a lying position on the side or stomach, to activate the muscles affecting the proprioceptors. Even if these exercises were effective, they would not be sufficient to meet the needs of the back. Unless you are under the age of 10, you typically spend most of your time sitting and standing. It is, therefore, essential to also do exercises that activate the muscles for posture and the proprioceptors, either in a standing or seated position.

Mastering Good Posture

Do you really want to give your back a treat? Try to master the following principles and your back will be deeply grateful.

Grounding

"Grounding" refers to having solid contact with the ground or floor and is essential for good posture. Without proper grounding, elongating the spinal column is basically useless and ineffective, since the spinal column has no solid base. Proper grounding requires the proprioceptors to work well. In everyday life, the two most important examples of grounding are:

- standing grounded (with only the feet);
- sitting grounded (with the pelvis and feet).

Standing Grounded

As we have seen in the inverted-pendulum model, small adjustments made by the feet have a major impact on the rest of the body. The feet must be rooted to the ground in order to achieve good posture. Weight must be divided evenly on both feet, and each foot must connect with the ground in a solid but relaxed fashion. To encourage grounding:

- **Spend part of each day in bare feet.** This will help you make a better connection with your feet when contacting the ground and will stimulate the proprioceptors and deep muscles in the feet. Keeping this in mind, it is not recommended that children constantly wear shoes in the early months of life. Feet develop better without shoes to support them. Constantly wearing shoes makes the feet, and indirectly the back, become dormant over time.

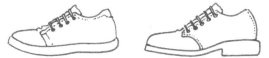

Neutral (flat) shoes

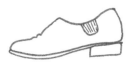

Low-heeled shoe

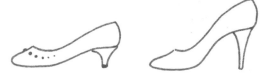

High-heeled shoes

Spinal Training Tip

To improve grounding, exercise number 2 (see page 109) is essential. It is one of the basic exercises to master in order to have a good back.

- **Your shoes must be as neutral (flat) as possible.** Avoid high heels. For walking or running, heels can be slightly raised, but for a stationary activity, it is better to wear shoes with a very low heel. In this way, the foot is activated in its natural position. A number of studies have shown links between wearing high heels and back problems.
- **Have a balanced base.** Our balance is dictated by our feet. Especially when handling a load, the stability of the balance base is provided by grounding. Depending on the activity, the spinal column should always remain above this base.

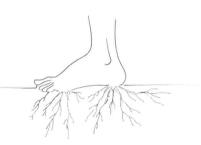

Grounded foot

Sitting Grounded

Because most of us spend more time sitting than standing, mastering the ability to sit grounded is essential. In front of the computer, feet have a tendency to move backward and lose contact with the floor. Once in a while, remind yourself to bring your feet forward and ground them properly. If you tend to cross your legs, you should know that this causes your pelvis to shift out of alignment. Your spinal column then has to compensate, causing a curvature in the spine. In the long run, this habit has a negative impact on posture. In addition, most people who cross their legs almost always do it on the same side, which causes more imbalance in the body.

Imagine that roots are growing out of your ischia (bones at the base of the pelvis) and will deeply anchor themselves in the seat of your chair and all the way down to the floor. This visual will guide you to ensure that the pelvis is well positioned to provide a solid base for your spinal column. Like a building, your spinal column cannot be properly erected if the foundation, in this case your pelvis, is not up to the task.

Positioning the pelvis is done in three steps:

- place your pelvis at the back of the seat;
- get your pelvis level by swiveling it into all corners of the seat;
- redistribute your weight evenly on the two ischia or the buttocks.

Ideally, we want a straight chair with a backrest that follows the spinal column.

Obviously we can't drag our ergonomic chair with us everywhere we go (imagine the burden!). But if you spend most of your time on one chair in particular (at work or at home), think of getting a chair that will be comfortable and help you achieve good posture effortlessly.

Therapeutic Advice

If your feet don't touch the floor, you won't be able to sit properly. In this case, place a footrest under your desk or at your workstation.

I'll admit, it is very difficult to maintain good sitting posture throughout an entire day. Don't feel guilty if you let go from time to time. Varying our posture helps to change the strain that is being put on the back. Here are several alternative positions to adopt.

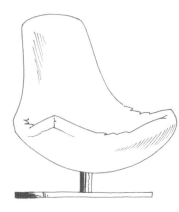

You'll have no end of trouble trying to achieve good posture in this modern-design chair that is not designed for proper back posture.

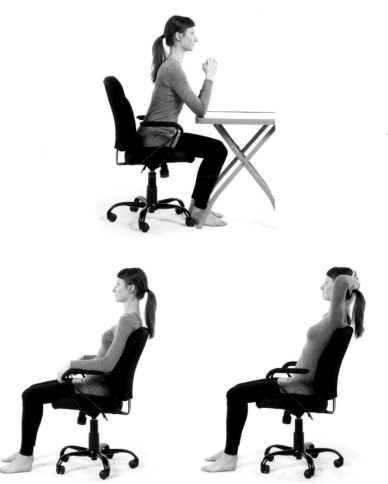

The sitting position also helps relax the muscles of the back and ease pain. Having the knees bent and legs raised is the position that places the least amount of stress on the back. While your back will benefit from rest periods, if you spend entire hours in this position, it will weaken your back in the long run.

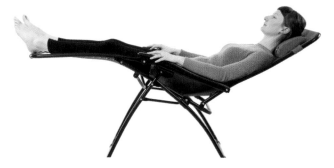

Elongation of the Spinal Column

There is no reason to put force on your lower back in order to sit up straight. Instead, work with your head.

Here are four easy steps to have a straight, elongated spinal column without effort.

1. Keep the Head Neutral

Maintain the head in a neutral position. No need to pull in or lift the chin. Look at the horizon.

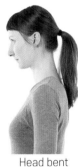 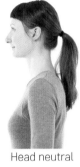 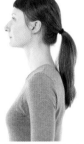

| Head bent | Head neutral | Head extended |

Therapeutic Advice

If you work at a computer, your screen should be adjusted to a height that allows you to maintain your head in this position. The most frequent error is to have a screen that is too low, which is always the case with laptop computers. Ensure that the height of the screen is at eye level.

2. Imagine a String at the Top of Your Skull

Visualize a little string attached to the top of your skull. Then, imagine that this string is slowly pulling your skull upward, without you having to make an effort.

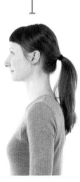

3. Lengthen the Neck

Next, imagine that your neck is slowly lengthening, without effort, like a cylinder that is regaining its normal shape. You, therefore, need to lengthen as much in the front (throat) as in the back (nape of the neck).

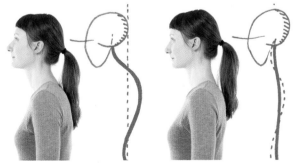

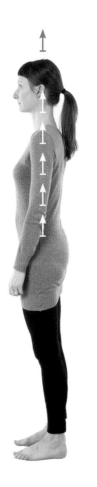

4. Lengthen the Entire Spinal Column

Finally, visualize your entire spinal column lengthening all the way down to the sacrum (base of the spinal column).

Starting with a slumped posture and applying this method, you can instantly take note of the lengthening without effort. Integrating these principles in everyday life does require some willpower. Besides, it's easier to slouch, but when you finally reap the rewards of your efforts, the work to engage your muscles will seem like a really small price to pay.

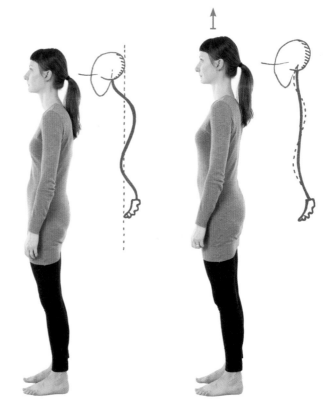

The Spinal Column at the Center

If I asked you to tell me if the spinal column is located in the front, center or back of the body, what would you answer? Most people have the impression that the spinal column is at the back of the body, which is explained by the fact that we can touch it easily only at the back. What we are actually touching, however, are the tips of the vertebrae's spiny apophyses. When we observe the position of the main part of the vertebrae and the disks, we discover that they are more in the center than we would have imagined. At the cervical and lumbar level, they are completely in the center of the body (unless one has a prominent belly). The thoracic region, however, needs to leave space for the lungs and heart, and so the spinal column is located farther back in that area. Nevertheless, it works in tandem with the ribs and sternum to form the chest. In looking at the entire chest, which functions as a unit, we realize that the spinal column is really in the center. It truly represents a central axis, much like the mast of a ship.

Myth No. 2: One Must Constantly Contract One's Abdominals

It is obvious that keeping one's abdominals contracted all day long and only relaxing them at night is a really bad idea. People contract their abdominals to appear slimmer and lift heavy objects. Doing this all day long, however, will add more pressure to the abdomen and pelvis, greatly reduce breathing, make organs less mobile and make the spinal column more rigid. To have a better silhouette, think about elongating the spinal column instead.

Respecting Curves

The spinal column, as you have probably noticed, is not straight. It includes curves, which are referred to as lordotic or kyphotic. Our spinal column, as suggested by its name, is like a Greek column, which is a stack of stable but heavy stones that are rigid and immobile. To perform all our movements, our spinal column has to be both mobile and stable. The curves give the spinal column suppleness, resistance and agility. It's a real triumph of engineering!

Elongating the spinal column should not be seen as eliminating curves, but regulating them. The ultimate objective is not to have a spinal column that is completely elongated and straight, but rather to allow the curves in the column to express themselves freely.

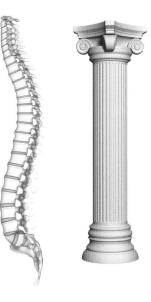

Seven Key Tips to Change Your Posture

1. Find the Posture that Suits You

As we read earlier, everyone has his or her own posture that is in part based on their genetic makeup. There is not one single model for posture. You must, therefore, find the posture that respects your back and suits you naturally. The key is to follow the principles of elongation and grounding, respecting the back's curves without trying to attain a perfectly straight ideal.

2. Make Changes

By improving your posture, even slightly, you will not only be giving your back a much-needed helping hand, but your relationship with your environment will also change. Need proof? Have a discussion with someone while your posture is slumped. After awhile, straighten up while continuing your conversation. You will notice that the dynamic will change between you and the person at the other end.

The change in posture will also change how you feel. Adopt a slumped posture for 30 minutes and chances are that you will feel lifeless. Then adopt a good posture for this same amount of time. You will notice that you have much more energy. There will be period of gradual adaptation before you see more permanent changes.

3. Use Little Effort

A little effort goes a long way to maintain good posture. You just need to know how to assume the right position. The deep muscles in the back will do the rest of the job. The trick is for the body to do this automatically.

In the early days in my rehabilitation practice, I often used the electromyogram (EMG), a test used to measure muscle contraction. This basically involves attaching sensors to muscles to record the intensity of a muscle contraction. The readings I obtained when someone was in a stationary standing position particularly stood out for me. The instrument indicated zero or very little muscle contraction in the superficial muscles. That's because the superficial muscles, those that are more apparent, are hardly used in a standing position. So then how does one stand upright? It's the fine and precise work of the small, deep muscles of the spinal column, and those of the lower limbs, that adjust constantly to keep us stable in space. If you assume the correct position, these muscles become more engaged and standing up straight requires little to no effort.

4. Relax

It is pointless to force an action. Relax the muscles that tend to be tensed: those of the jaws, the face, the muscles between the eyes, the shoulder muscles and the muscles of the pelvic floor.

5. Work in An Ergonomic Way

Ergonomics take into account the characteristics of a person, such as average height or the length of their stride, that need to be considered in designing a space in which they work or spend a lot of time. For example, worktables might be designed higher in university than in elementary school or steps in public spaces might be built lower in Asia to accommodate a shorter population. Individuals who are not of average height can have difficulty finding a suitable working environment. It often happens that a short person at a standard workstation cannot even place her feet on the floor. At the flip side, a strapping fellow of 6 ft. 4 in. (1.95 m) will have to bend over most work surfaces.

Ergonomics is particularly important in a sitting position given the number of hours most people spend this way. If your chair has a rounded back or your desk is too low, it will be difficult for you to adopt good posture. In the standing position, it is easier to compensate using one's legs. Let's take our tall fellow, who is a cook, and place him at a low worktable to chop 20 onions.

The worktable is set up for a person measuring a height of 5 ft. 8 in. (1.75 m). To avoid weeping for reasons other than the allyl sulfates from the onion, he can spread his feet and bend his knees to position himself at a better height for his back, or better yet, adjust the worktable to a suitable height for himself. A small adjustment can have a major impact.

6. Be Aware of Your Body

Not everyone is fully aware of his or her body. Some people who are more kinesthetic, such as professional dancers, have precise awareness. Others who lack this awareness may have a great deal of difficulty describing a pain and even locating it. When you have a low level of body awareness you tend to be more attracted to vigorous exercises because they accentuate the muscles that are being worked. People with a high level of body awareness are more comfortable with relaxation, breathing and posture exercises because they have a better sense of how their body is reacting to them. Follow your nature and choose the exercises that suit you.

7. Give Yourself Time

If your posture has been slumped for years, your deep muscles have become used to doing very little and are probably weakened. Give them time to awaken and strengthen. The first attempts might bring on a lot of stiffness, as your deep muscles make their appearance and protest loudly. On average, you should count on:

- one week to awaken and sense the deep muscles;
- two weeks to sense a change in posture;
- one month to obtain lasting changes.

Improving Your Body Awareness

- Have a better understanding of your body (this is one of the book's objectives).
- Visualize your body and the zones that are activated during an exercise. For example, to engage your abdominal muscles, visualize an internal lumbar support belt made up of your deep abdominal muscles.
- Do exercises from time to time that require you to listen to your body (breathing, posture, flexibility, neuromuscular relaxation, etc.)
- Accept your limits. Do not try to achieve the maximum at all costs. During a stretching exercise, for example, it does no good to strain your body to the limit with a grimace.
- Relax the muscles that are not being used. Your jaw will not help your hands to lift a weight and your forehead muscles will not increase the power in your thighs!
- Be conscious of your alignment during your movements.

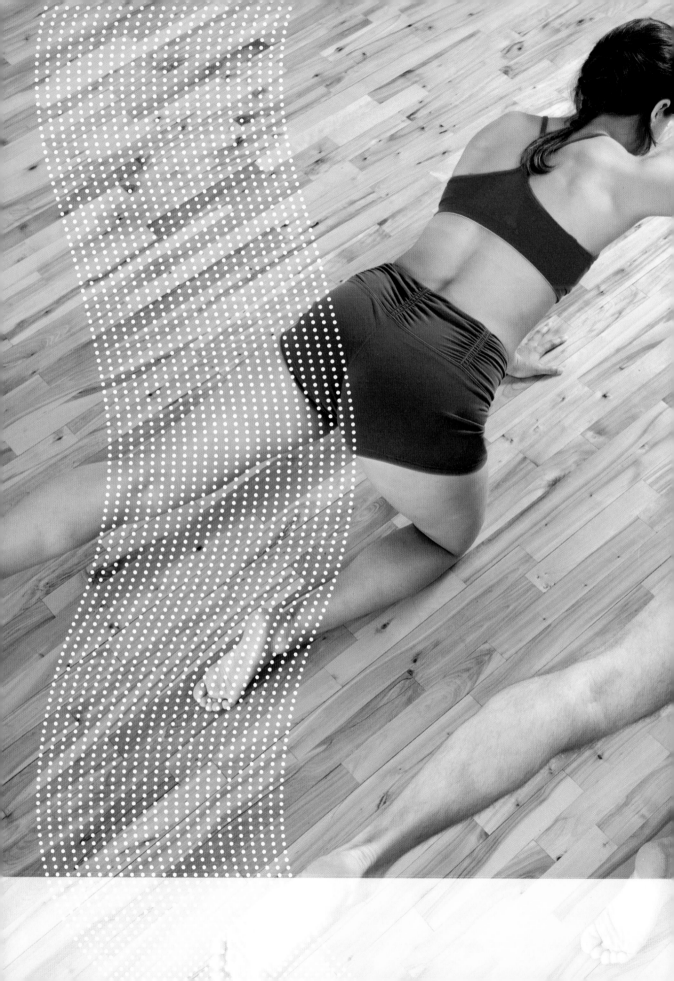

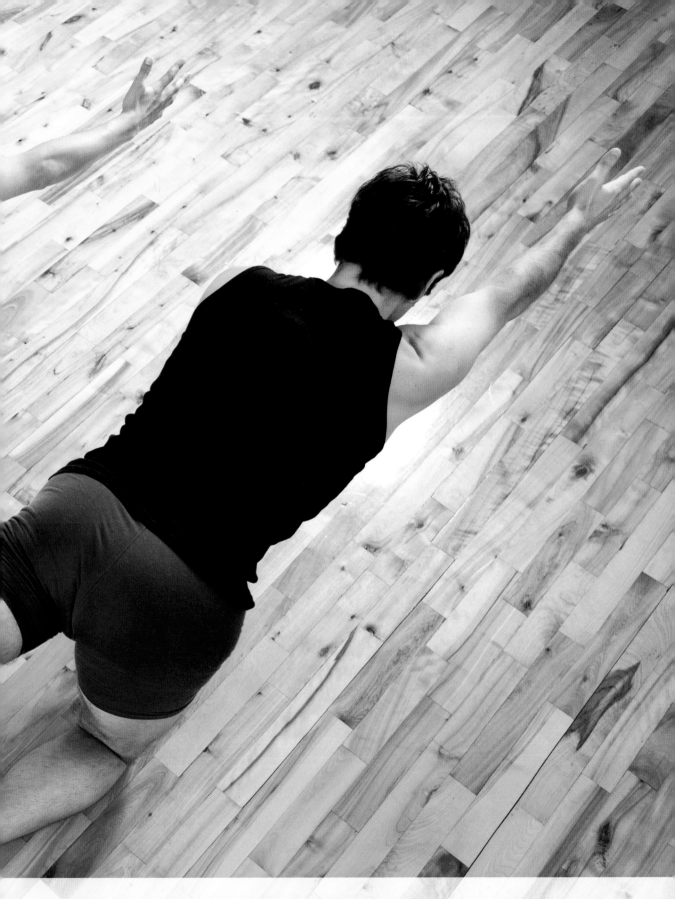

CHAPTER 4: A BACK IN MOTION

The Body Strives to Be Healthy

With all the stories we hear today about people afflicted with disease (cancer, irritable bowel syndrome, diabetes, high blood pressure, hypothyroidism, stroke, herniated disk, etc.), it's normal to be concerned about our own health. If you're worried sick over the hundreds of diseases and conditions that could strike, remember this: the body naturally strives to be healthy, not ill. I often repeat this bit of inspiration to my patients (and to myself). Remember, too, that the body is designed to self-regulate, as long as we take good care of it.

Self-Regulation

At every moment, without thinking about it, your body's regulatory systems send out a formidable battalion to regenerate your organs, muscles, bones and nerves, fight viruses and bacteria, control your breathing, digestion and elimination, and more.

The nervous, hormonal and immune systems work to keep your body stable (homeostasis) through a complex set of internal mechanisms. With this in mind, you may be surprised that a physical therapist will tell you that no therapist can heal a patient. The therapist does play a part in the process of healing — for example, by providing treatment to help restore mobility to a patient's lumbar vertebrae. This, in turn, helps the patient's natural mechanisms regain their ability to self-regulate. In short, the therapist frees the patient's body from constraints that are preventing him from regulating his own systems.

Physical training, done correctly and in the right dose, also helps improve the function of the body's regulatory systems. It has a direct effect on the body's ability to self-regulate. It is a known fact that elite athletes have a better immune system and a more effective nervous system, along with a better ability to recover. In the case of excessive training, where it is too intense or prolonged without sufficient recovery time, however, we see the opposite. We all have the tools within us to be healthy. All we need to do is activate them by moving our bodies.

> We all have the tools within us to be healthy. All we need to do is to activate them by moving our bodies.

Adaptation

Along with self-regulation, the body has the ability to adapt to whatever stress it is facing. Luckily for us, unless the stress is too repetitive, our body adapts and becomes more resistant to stress. In this way, through properly supervised training, we get into better physical condition. The exercises in this book will help your body adapt by improving your posture, increasing muscle endurance in your back and improving the function of your diaphragm so that you breathe more easily, among others. With training, we can even develop our sense of taste and smell (think of oenologists), the voice (singers), the sense of touch (the blind who learn to read Braille), etc. In short, everyone can adapt and improve.

But the ability to adapt is a double-edged sword. If the body is never subjected to any stress, it adapts by becoming less resistant to stress. Let's take the example of astronauts after a space mission. Their bone density has diminished so much that they need to follow a physical training program upon their return. When one is no longer subjected to gravity for a prolonged period, the need for the body to have strong bones is eliminated. If we examine the way we live today, we see a similar recurrence affecting the body.

Spinal Training Tip

The objective of Spinal Training is to relaunch these two mechanisms — self-regulation and adaption — for a strong back and an iron constitution.

As we become less active and spend more time sitting, our body is becoming accustomed to doing nothing, and our back is becoming less supple and resistant. Spinal Training sends the right signals to the back so that it can adapt in the best way possible.

You Decide

☐ I will let my body become accustomed to doing nothing.

OR

☐ I will help my body adapt to movement.

What Are the Objectives of Back Exercises?

Responding to the Back's Requirements

Being constantly bombarded by infomercials and advertisements extolling the virtues of having sculpted abs of steel and a powerful back, we lose sight of what our back really needs.

If your spinal column could talk, it would say: I need…

- good mobility between my vertebrae;
- suppleness in my muscles;
- relaxation;
- strength in my deep muscles;
- good posture;
- more energy.

The best way to respond to your back's requirements is to answer, I do the following:

- flexibility exercises;
- mobility exercises;
- neuromuscular relaxation and breathing exercises;
- deep muscle strengthening exercises;
- postural exercises;
- cardiovascular exercises.

Satisfy the needs of your spinal column and it will be happy. The objective of Spinal Training is to respond to all these needs in the best way possible. Most people don't really know how to take care of their back, and even when they rely on a physical trainer or group instructor, they may not be well informed. Whether you have a personal trainer or group instructor, it is essential that you ensure they have the appropriate skills to guide you properly. Look for a trainer with a recognized diploma who regularly updates his or her skills through ongoing training in the area of back problems. You owe it to yourself and your back.

Protecting Your Back

To protect your back, core-strengthening exercises are the first line of defense, and do much more for you than a lumbar support belt could. If your core muscles function well, stress is distributed equally throughout your body, relieving pressure from your spinal column. Let's take the example of weight lifters. With very strong core muscles, they can lift weights that, according to biomechanical calculations, would normally cause serious damage to their spinal column, intervertebral disks and other areas of the back.

Another way to protect your back is to know how to handle loads. You need strong legs and training to develop this skill. Having the right posture, another skill you learn in training, helps diminish the stress placed on your back and protect it over the long term.

Paradoxically, while good training helps protect the back, some exercises have the opposite effect. A number of studies have shown that too much stress is placed on the back during many common exercises (see the following section). They should be avoided, even if they seem very attractive ("What a beautiful pose!") or effective ("It looks like you really work out hard!"). Respect your back and it will reward you generously.

Myth No. 4: The Latest Ab Super Machine Will Change Your Life!

Like me, in a moment of weakness, you may have succumbed to one of these infomercials touting the benefits of some revolutionary training device. These devices have remained popular since the late 1980s, promising us sculpted abs and a substantial reduction in our waistline in less than four weeks, all thanks to a device that fits under the bed! No study has been done on the extended use of these gadgets, but my hunch is that these devices most often remain under the bed. What's more, if we trust the testimonials with the before and after photos, we would note that these devices also seem to tan skin and whiten teeth!

In fact, no training aimed solely at strengthening abdominals can help the back or be associated with the loss of abdominal fat. An exercise can improve the muscle tone of the targeted zone, but cannot have an impact on one's fat reserves. It is the same for fat in the thighs, better known as "saddlebags." It's just not possible to have a Hollywood-star figure and a spine of steel in less than three minutes a day. You don't need any equipment to help your back. The most sophisticated equipment by far is your back itself, and the only cost is the time you spend looking after it.

Exercises to Avoid

These exercises can be harmful to your back. Some people may not agree with this list, having decided that a certain exercise is doing them a lot of good. While that may be possible, each person has his or her own needs and perhaps a particular condition they're living with. The list that follows considers two main questions:

- Does the exercise meet the back's requirements and respect its natural movements? If the answer is no, the exercise will not serve a purpose, unless you are a circus acrobat.
- Can the exercise cause back problems? If the answer is yes, it should be absolutely avoided. As a physical therapist and trainer, I have observed many problems caused by the following exercises.

Abdominal Strengthening Exercises

The following exercises put a lot of pressure on the lower back. They are an excellent way to damage your disks. They more often activate the hip flexors (iliopsoas) than the abdominals, and can be dangerous for people with back problems. Stop doing them immediately. They will do your back more harm than good.

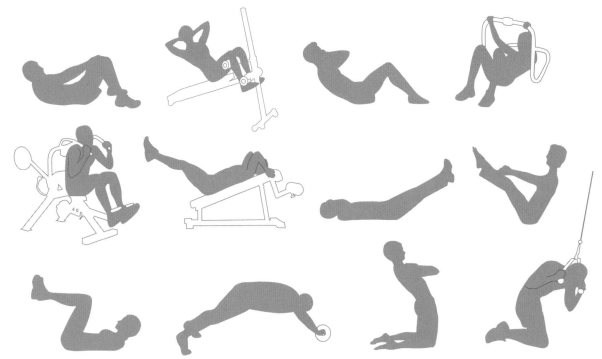

Back Strengthening Exercises

These exercises are too restrictive for the spinal column. For most people, the pressure exerted exceeds the resistance of the spinal column. These exercises do not meet the natural requirements of the back muscles, that is to say, they do not help to make the slight adjustments that are needed to achieve good posture. Unless you are a weight lifter, avoid them.

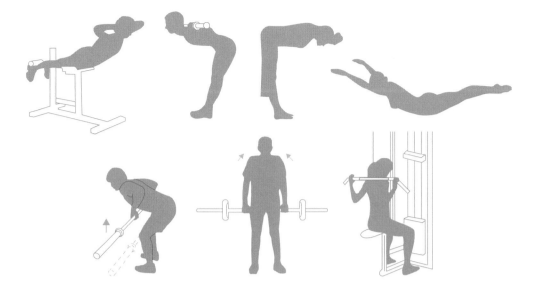

Extreme Poses

For most people, the following poses do not respect the spinal column's mobility or resistance. Unless one is especially supple, stable and able to perfectly master these poses after a long and slow progression, they are risky. I can't even count the number of yoga instructors who come to me with severe back problems as a result of doing these poses repeatedly.

Headstand Poses

Headstand poses can take years to fully master. They are an integral part of some forms of yoga training and can be beneficial to one's health. Two main issues, however, pose a problem. First, when we study the mechanics of the spinal column, we discover that it is not at all adapted to this type of pose. The first two vertebrae of the neck (atlas and axis) and the vertebrae in general are not designed to support significant weight in a position that is opposite to what is natural. Second, even if the pressure put on the head is diminished by good support on the forearms, the risk of injury remains high, due to the difficulty of maintaining this pose in a well-controlled manner. The risk that is taken is, therefore, too great for the potential benefits.

Inverted Poses

These poses place a lot of stress on the junction between the neck and the chest. Bending at this point is not natural and is risky if the movement is not perfectly controlled.

Extreme Stretch Poses

These poses require a level of mobility in the back that many people do not have. They represent a risk of serious injury. Unless you are a circus acrobat, avoid them. The only exception is the traditional cobra pose (top-left image). This pose can be effective, provided it is done very gradually, by leaving the forearms on the ground, for example, not arching the back too much and by contracting the core muscles.

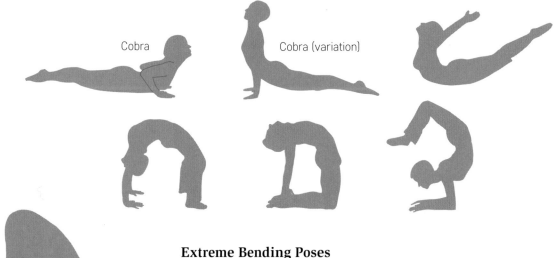

Cobra

Cobra (variation)

Extreme Bending Poses

Standing poses with the trunk bent forward are suitable for people with good flexibility and a healthy back. Otherwise, it is better to avoid this type of exercise, as a lot of pressure is put on the disks. It is preferable to do stretches that are effective but still safe. People who are dealing with a herniated disc are strictly advised not to do this type of exercise.

Best Exercises for Your Back

When it comes to finding consensus on the best exercises for the back, there are several currents of thought that seem to contradict one another. According to one of them, flexibility exercises are the key. As a result, muscle strengthening is completely eliminated from certain training methods. At the opposite end, another view says that exercises to strengthen and stabilize the body are key, thus totally eliminating flexibility exercises. Yet another mind-set maintains that everything can be regulated through breathing and relaxation exercises. Without going into the details of all the principal approaches, it is rare to find a method that takes into account the back's and the body's full requirements. The objective of Spinal Training is to meet these requirements in a way that will improve the back on all levels.

The Spinal Training Approach

Spinal Training targets seven different and complementary parameters in order to meet the back's requirements. Each of these parameters is essential and requires proper training, and has an influence on other parameters. For example, if you are not flexible, this will affect your muscle strength, the mobility in your spinal column, your breathing, the equilibrium of your nervous system and more.

The Seven Parameters of Spinal Training

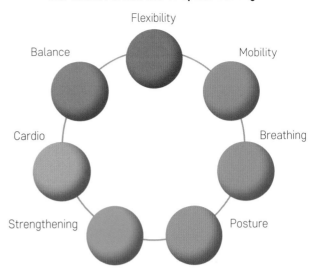

Spinal Training Vs. Classic Models

The Conventional Approach in the Gym

For years, the conventional training in most gyms has consisted of cardio, followed by muscle strengthening and ending with a short stretching routine.

Most of the parameters are left out in this approach. The strengthening exercises most often focus on the superficial muscles and are not sufficiently targeted to the back.

Flexibility	✓
Mobility	✗
Breathing	✗
Posture	✗
Strengthening	✗
Cardio	✓
Balance	✓

3/7

The Approach Centered on Flexibility

Full stretching sessions that are properly executed help improve breathing and back mobility. They also help rebalance the nervous system, and thus are very beneficial to the back. Stretching on its own, however, won't create good posture, provide adequate cardio or help develop effective deep muscles.

Flexibility	✓
Mobility	✓
Breathing	✓
Posture	✗
Strengthening	✗
Cardio	✗
Balance	✓

4/7

The Approach Centered on Strengthening

The people who are double-jointed are those who can most benefit from training that is centered uniquely on strengthening. Otherwise, this approach is very limited.

Flexibility	✗
Mobility	✗
Breathing	✗
Posture	✗
Strengthening	✓
Cardio	✗
Balance	✗

1/7

These equal a happy back in a healthy body!

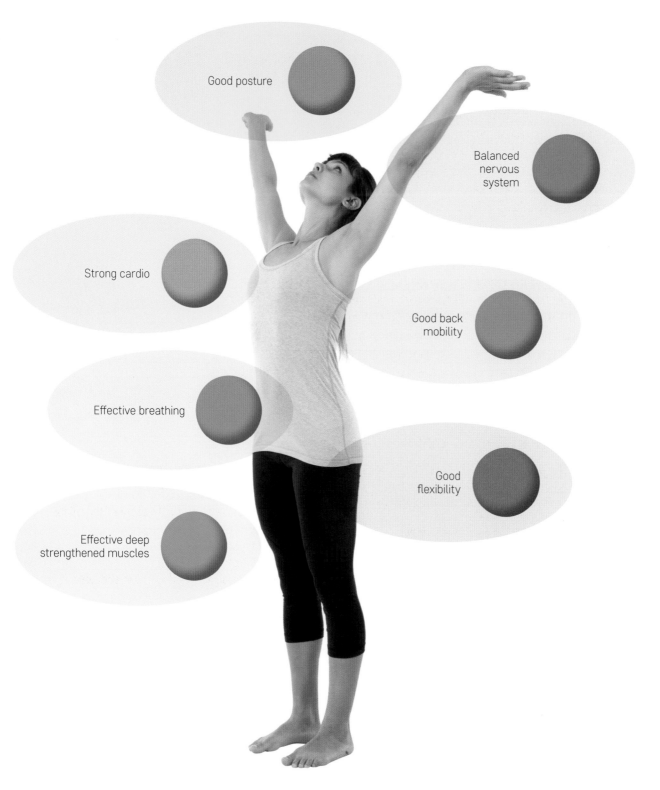

Good posture

Balanced nervous system

Strong cardio

Good back mobility

Effective breathing

Good flexibility

Effective deep strengthened muscles

Components of Spinal Training

1. Flexibility Exercises

Flexibility exercises (also called stretches) are one of the best ways to rebalance the back before adding other elements to the program. We all know that stretching helps improve the suppleness of muscles. This type of exercise also has an impact on fascia (the layer of connective tissue that envelops the muscles) and even the nerves. Fascia is what binds the muscles together in muscular chains. Picture the almost transparent membrane covering a chicken breast, or imagine several layers of plastic wrap bound together and connecting the muscles, bones, organs and nervous system. It is only in the anatomy books that you find isolated muscles. We never stretch one single muscle, but a muscular chain.

What Muscles Should Be Stretched?

Now that you know that the body is made up of muscular chains, you may be wondering which muscles or muscular chains really need to be stretched. Should the entire body be stretched? According to the theories of Dr. Vladimir Janda, certain muscles (said to be "tonic") are inclined to stretch and other muscles (said to be "phasic") are weak. Tonic muscles must be stretched first.

In the flexibility exercise section (see page 114), you will find effective exercises that target the tonic muscles. Optimal results are achieved by knowing which muscles to stretch.

Spinal Training Tip

Spinal Training takes this difference into account, working to stretch the muscles that are inclined to be stretched and strengthen the muscles that are inclined to be weak. Therefore, it's incorrect to think that we need to stretch and strengthen all the muscles of the body.

The Principal Tonic and Phasic Muscles*

Tonic muscles (which are inclined to stretch)	Phasic muscles (which are inclined to weaken)
• Hamstring (back of the thigh)	• Vastus medialis and lateralis (front of the thigh)
• Calves (especially the deep layers)	• Interior tibialis (front of the leg)
• Lumbar spinal	• Rectus abdominis muscle
• Cervical spinal	• Flexor muscles of the neck
• Pectoral	• Rhomboid muscles (between the shoulder blades)
• Deep gluteal	• Gluteus maximus (superficial part)
• Large dorsal	• Triceps
• Quadratus lumborum	• Lower and middle trapezius
• Upper trapezius	
• Iliopsoas	
• Jaw	

* according to Dr. Vladimir Janda

Flexibility and the Nervous System

Flexibility exercises not only help to make the muscles more supple, but they also have a little known effect on the back: they help the nervous system achieve equilibrium. The effect of stretching, then, has a major impact on one of the body's regulatory systems, the nervous system. How is that possible? When it is unbalanced by one factor or another (emotional stress, physical fatigue, digestive issue, back problem, etc.), the nervous system increases the tonicity in certain muscles said to be tonic. By stretching them, their tonicity diminishes, which helps the nervous system to rebalance. The next time you do a flexibility exercise, remember that you are also giving your nervous system a precious helping hand.

Spinal Training Tip

Do mobility exercises that are equivalent to oiling and scraping the rust from each of the joints in the spinal column so that it can better express itself.

2. Mobility Exercises

Mobility exercises, along with stretching, are one of the best starting points for restoring your back to health. Mobility refers to movement in the joints (between the vertebrae, in the knees, ankles, hips, shoulders, jaw, etc.). In the spinal column, it is essential to have good mobility between each vertebra. It is also important in the pelvis and the chest (the ribs are connected to the vertebrae). Ultimately, one needs to have good mobility in all the joints. A rigid ankle, knee or hip can change one's gait and affect the back. Even stiffness in a shoulder, elbow or forearm can have an impact on the back because of its connection to the shoulder blades and the spinal column. If your spinal column is as stiff as an iron rod or your chest is as rigid as a steel drum, strengthening exercises will only accentuate the problem. You need to begin by improving your mobility. Take the example of a leg that is set in a cast for four weeks. The cast prevents any mobility. This results in muscular atrophy (loss of muscle) and poorer circulation. The same phenomenon occurs in a joint that is not mobile, such as when there is a vertebral blockage.

Finally, the sitting posture diminishes mobility in the back. It will do you no good to spend the day sitting and then doing sit-ups. You have to get your back moving. A mobile back is a back for life!

3. Breathing Exercises

We start breathing a few seconds after birth and maintain this essential action until the very end. We breathe about 20,000 times a day, and each time the back is put in motion. The thoracic diaphragm is the main muscle responsible for breathing. It alone works to ensure normal breathing. As it contracts, it helps expand the rib cage, creating more space in the lungs by lowering the pressure inside them. The air thus automatically enters the lungs. When exhaling, the diaphragm relaxes and the air is expelled naturally from the lungs. When we make an effort (even when we rest), that is, if we are having difficulty breathing, our other muscles move into action.

The diaphragm has the special ability to contract both involuntarily and voluntarily. When you try to contract the diaphragm voluntarily, something interesting takes place. Let's try this experiment together. If you are sitting, assume an upright posture that is as comfortable as possible. Now, just try to breathe for one minute, allowing the stomach to expand.

What do you feel? If you recognize the sensations described in the table below, try the suggested solutions. You will definitely benefit from breathing exercises.

SENSATION	SOLUTION
It's really a challenge to breathe this way.	You need to train your breathing.
It's difficult to remain sitting up straight.	You need to train your posture.
That was a very long minute.	You need to relax.
My chest feels tight, as though it's preventing me from breathing freely.	You need to do mobility exercises.
I wonder if I just got another e-mail.	You need to switch off!

4. Posture Exercises

Now you know more about posture and how training the posture muscles and proprioceptors is one of the keys to having a good back.

The posture exercises have an advantage because they're easy to do in all kinds of situations. Here are a few examples:

Standing

- in a waiting line;
- on the bus;
- at the airport;
- in the subway.

Sitting

- during a course;
- during a break, in front of the computer;
- waiting for someone at a restaurant;
- during a commercial.

Antigravity Devices

Some people praise the virtues of antigravity devices, which are designed to ease back pain and regulate back problems. The cost of treatments that use this equipment is usually high. These devices are supposed to relieve the disks from the pressures of evil gravity. In reality, these devices do nothing to eliminate the problem, which is not gravity, as we read earlier. Imagine that your body finds itself weightless for a while. It's possible you will feel relief, but when you return to the normal world, your body is once again subjected to the force of gravity and the relief will be short-lived if your body has lost the habit of functioning in this environment. You should, therefore, choose exercises and postures that will help you work with gravity, rather than using devices designed to remove you from it. Save your money on unproven gadgets and, instead, concentrate on better posture and exercises that meet your back's requirements.

Helical Elongations: A New Way to Improve Posture

After years of research, with the objective of finding the best way to train the deep muscles of the spinal column and improve posture, I developed some very special exercises called helical elongations. These exercises should be done in a standing position and can be transposed into everyday movements. Starting with the image of uncorking a bottle of champagne (you will soon understand), I experimented with helical elongations (or helicals, for simplicity's sake) for several months, and the results were very interesting. I began recommending the exercises to professional dancers and elite athletes, with very positive results. Better posture, diminished back pain, the sensation of being taller and having more control over one's spinal column — just some of the feedback I received. Helicals have since become an integral part of Spinal Training and many people consider them one of its essential components.

Given these results, I started to recommend helicals to my patients. While most of them had some difficulty with the subtle nature of helicals at the beginning, in fairly short order they made excellent progress.

What Are Helicals?

The term "helical" refers to a lengthening movement in the spinal column combined with a spiral movement, reminiscent of a corkscrew in action. Several kinds of helical forms are found in nature. Think of the double helix that makes up our DNA chain, certain viruses or the well-known *helicobacter pylori* (H. pylori) bacteria that cause most stomach ulcers. But let's get back to our corkscrew. Imagine that your spinal column is a long champagne cork, and that your legs and pelvis are the bottle of champagne. Your cork is firmly compressed into your bottle. Imagine that you want to pull this cork out of the bottle. If you have ever removed a champagne cork, you know that the best way to do it is to pull upward (elongation) and turn (helical). That's a helical elongation! The idea is to open up your spinal column in the same way that one pulls on a champagne cork, turning one way and then the other. You will notice that there is no pop or explosion of fizzy liquid to accompany this helical elongation.

5. Strengthening Exercises

Muscle strengthening is an important part of Spinal Training. At the same time, good mobility and good flexibility in the spinal column are also crucial. Strengthening exercises are added gradually to the routines as the level of difficulty increases. A common mistake is to add in the strengthening exercises with unbalanced posture and a spinal column that is not very mobile, only to find that you are even more unbalanced or in pain after a few weeks.

The core muscles and the muscles of the central axis are the most important and the first to be activated, for four main reasons:

- they are responsible for posture;
- if the core muscles are more stable and mobile, peripheral movements can be made more freely and efficiently;
- when they don't work in the right way, they can be responsible for vertebral blockages because of their direct attachment to the vertebrae;
- they are often responsible for back pain.

One can then target the postural muscles of the lower limbs, the superficial muscles in the trunk, and finally, those of the arms. There is no point developing muscles in your biceps and your pectorals before adequately training the deep muscles in your back. Your limbs will be stronger if you are supported with solid core muscles.

The Core Muscles and the Muscles of the Central Axis

The diagrams on the next page will help you better visualize the muscles that need to be trained. You can also review the anatomical charts on pages 24 and 25 for more accurate information on the different muscles being used.

Core Muscles

A — The Deep Abdominals and the Quadratus Lumborum Muscle
Start by visualizing a cylinder that wraps around the entire abdomen. This cylinder, or core, mainly consists of deep abdominal muscles. They are completed by the quadratus lumborum and rectus abdominis muscles (superficial abdominal muscles).

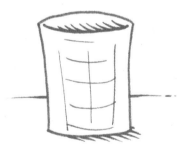

A1 — Transversus Abdominis Muscle
The deepest layer in the abdominals is the transversus abdominis muscle. It's one of the key muscles for the back. It protects the back like a lumbar support belt, but much more effectively. Its horizontal muscle fibers wrap around the abdomen and attach to the lumbar spinal column (in the lower back).

Myth No. 5: Strong Abdominals = A Good Back

For a few decades, sit-ups have been the gold standard exercise, followed closely by the familiar push-ups. But it is time we change our way of thinking. You do need strong abdominals, and in cases where you do, these are limited. Sit-ups should not be done any which way. Conventional sit-ups only work the superficial layer of the abdominals (the much sought-after "six-pack") and the psoas muscles, which serve no purpose being strengthened among the general population. Abdominal muscles are not activated unless you do it voluntarily (you will soon learn how). Sit-ups, therefore, are of very little use to the back unless you are an acrobat, professional dancer or elite athlete. Even if that were the case, you still need to strengthen the deep abdominal muscles before thinking of strengthening the superficial abdominal muscles.

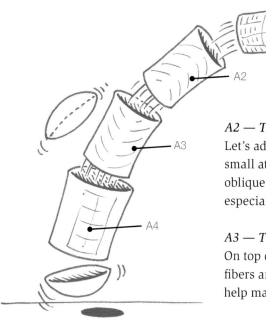

A2 — The Internal Oblique Muscle

Let's add a layer that partially envelops the abdomen, with small attachments to the lower back: these are the internal oblique muscles. Their fibers are arranged diagonally and are especially active during twisting movements.

A3 — The External Oblique Muscle

On top of this, let's add another layer of oblique muscles whose fibers are also arranged diagonally in the opposite direction, to help make the abdomen more firm.

A4 — The Rectus Abdominis Muscle

On this already well-equipped belt, let's superimpose a layer in front: the rectus abdominis muscle. This is the most visible muscle as it is the most superficial one. It is the muscle that many people work out in the hope of obtaining a developed and sculpted abdomen.

A5 — The Quadratus Lumborum Muscle

To complete the set, let's add the quadratus lumborum muscles in back. They attach directly to the vertebrae of the lower back and are useful in movements that require the back to lean.

B — The Pelvic Floor and the Piriformis Muscle

Next, under this cylinder, let's add a half-sphere that encloses the pelvis from underneath.

B1 — Pelvic Floor Muscle

The pelvic floor is one of the most important muscles in the back. It controls pressure in the pelvis and must contract each time you contract your abdominals. Without it, the organs in the pelvis (bladder, uterus or prostate, rectum) would be pulled toward the ground. The pelvic floor (which includes the perineum in women) almost single-handedly encloses the pelvis.

B2 — Piriformis Muscles

The piriformis muscles, once referred to as "pyramidals," close up the space that is not filled by the pelvic floor. These muscles are often tense and can be a source of irritation in the sciatic nerve, which passes under the piriformis muscles, or in some cases, through them.

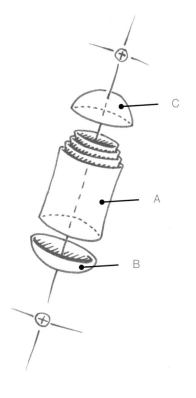

Myth No. 6: A Strong Back = A Healthy Back

Many trainers recommend strengthening the muscles of the back to prevent back problems. In reality, this is more likely to attract back problems. Strengthening gradually affects the superficial muscles (large dorsal, trapezius, etc.) but not the deep muscles of the spinal column. Moreover, these superficial back muscles are often tense. They need to be stretched and not subjected to heavy muscle building. Most of all, the back requires its deep muscles to work effectively. These thin, small muscles only need to be slightly contracted over a long period of time. Again, for certain sports, physical labor or activities, it is a good idea to develop the superficial muscles in a specific way, but only once the deep muscles are working effectively. As a physical therapist and a trainer, I've seen many people injure their backs doing strengthening exercises, usually at a gym.

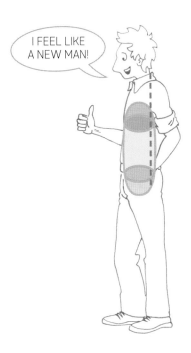

I FEEL LIKE A NEW MAN!

C — The Thoracic Diaphragm

Let's complete our first part of the diagram with a half-sphere (or dome) that encloses the top part. This is the thoracic diaphragm, which is the muscle for breathing.

D — The Deep Muscles of the Spinal Column

The deep muscles start at the base of the skull and go all the way down to the sacrum, attaching to the vertebrae in succession (the deepest level) or the ribs. They are thin, small muscles that are too deep to be apparent.

Endurance vs. Power

The word "strengthening" can be confused with muscle strength training. In reality, the deep muscles need to have more endurance.

Unless you are a weight lifter or elite athlete who has to make intense efforts, your back works mainly with endurance. For this reason, it is not very useful to do exercises with heavy weights. You also risk injuring yourself.

TARGETED TRAINING	EFFORT	DURATION	EXAMPLE OF ACTIVITY
Endurance	Light	Long	Sitting or standing posture, walking, running, etc.
Resistance	Moderate	Medium	Series of muscle-building exercises (10 to 15 repetitions)
Strength	Intense	Short	• Series of muscle-building exercises (1 to 6 repetitions) with a heavy load • Lifting a very heavy object
Power	Intense and rapid	Short	Weight lifting

6. Cardiovascular Exercises

The impact of cardiovascular training (called "cardio" here for short) is greatly underestimated. It is one of the training parameters for any situation. The effects of cardio are too great to ignore, including:

- lowered or stabilized blood pressure;
- improvement in cardiovascular capacity;
- lowered heartbeat at rest;
- greater endurance when making an effort;
- improved immune system;
- weight loss or weight maintenance;
- better digestion;
- better mood;
- more restorative sleep.

All of these effects have a positive impact on the back. Weight loss combined with cardio training reduces strain on the back, better sleep helps the nervous system recover, the back (through its connection to the nervous system) is consequently more relaxed and functional, and the more general effects of cardio help the back to express itself normally, thus improving the body's physiology.

Some cardiovascular exercises are better than others for the back. Running, for example, is more useful than cycling. In this case, we aren't talking about the pleasure of doing an activity, but the activation of the muscles of the back and proprioceptors. The best activities are done in a relatively natural standing position, whether it is in running shoes or on a snowboard.

Don't deprive yourself of cardio training that makes you happy and suits you on the pretext that it is less beneficial for the back. There will always be more positive effects than negative effects. The question is whether you always do the same kind of cardio training. A person who always trains on a bicycle and spends the rest of his time sitting does not really help his back. While swimming is a great physical activity, and some people really benefit from it, a person who only swims for physical activity never helps her body adapt to gravity in her training. If that's your case, make sure you combine your training with other activities, such as strengthening or postural exercises.

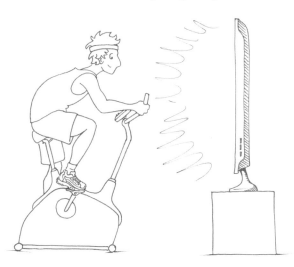

Exercises that Greatly Benefit the Back

- walking, hiking
- running
- cross-country skiing
- snowshoeing
- tennis
- soccer
- basketball, handball, volleyball
- dancing

Myth No. 7: Running Is Bad for the Back

As an instructor in biomechanics who has been running more or less regularly for 30 years, my hair stands on end when I hear this remark. In the 1990s, word got around that running leads to back and knee problems. People were advised to walk instead of running and were told that walking is healthier. In fact, studies have shown that runners do not have more back or knee problems than non-runners. On the contrary, running is one of the best exercises for the back. The back has had time to adapt since man started running some 2.5 million years ago! The problem is that our back has developed the habit of not doing anything. Consequently, if we don't start running gradually, we may experience pain all over, as well as in the back. By doing Spinal Training, anyone (except in special circumstances) who moves gradually and listens to his or her body, can manage to run. If you want to lose weight, running is one of the best exercises.

Exercises that Are Somewhat Beneficial for the Back

- cycling
- swimming
- inline or ice skating
- rowing
- kayaking
- canoeing

Spinal Training Tip

You can apply the principles of Spinal Training to cardio, making your workout even more effective.

Training the Back with Cardio

Cardio training takes into account your heart rate, the duration of exercise, intensity of effort and the number of training sessions a week. Proper cardio training is a science in itself. However, little is known about the quality of movement and posture. These elements are very important and have a bearing on whether cardio training will be beneficial or harmful to your back. Here are key areas to activate when you're doing cardio. In this chart, they are applied to walking and running.

TARGET AREAS	IN RUNNING OR WALKING
Posture	• The spinal column should remain elongated. • The feet should be solid on the ground.
Breathing	• It should be full and deep.
Core muscles	• They should be slightly activated.
Muscle relaxation	• The shoulders, jaw, arms, hands and face should be relaxed. • Avoid unnecessary tension.
Mobility	• With the help of the arms, the trunk should turn freely toward the opposite hip with each stride. • Movement should be done smoothly and easily.

Two Effective Ways To Do Cardio Training

- **Endurance training:** The goal here is to increase the duration of the training in order to tire the body, which will respond by developing endurance. Aim for low- to medium-intensity effort. You should be able to hold a conversation during the activity.

The activity's duration should be a minimum of 30 minutes and can go up to an hour-plus.

- **Interval training:** This type of training alternates low- and high-intensity effort. Endurance athletes typically follow such programs. Although specialists consider this the most effective type of cardio training, it must be done in the right dose and respect the back's limitation. If an increased heartbeat is the objective, the mechanics must follow accordingly — the heart and lungs can't work properly unless the back is able to withstand the intense effort of running fast and impact with each step. I can't count the number of the athletes who have come to see me with back pain following high-intensity training. I suggest increasing the intensity gradually so your body's mechanisms have time to adapt.

Here are two suggestions for effective training:

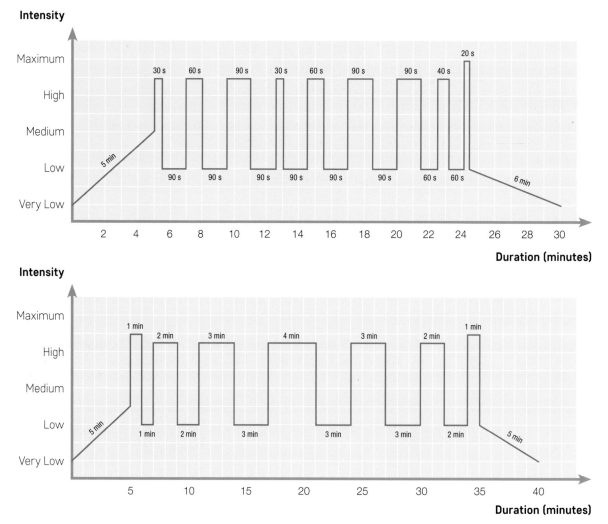

The Importance of Walking

Even though walking does not increase your heartbeat in a significant way (making it less interesting for developing cardio), it remains a basic activity for the back and, in general, for maintaining health. Among other things, it helps activate the deep muscles of the back, mobilize the spinal column, stimulate the diaphragm and relax the body and mind. For our famous *homo sittingus*, it represents a first step on the road to good health.

7. Balance Exercises

Here, the term "balance" refers to balancing the nervous system. Yes, that's right, one of the benefits of training with balance exercises, in general, is to help rebalance the nervous system, which is inseparable from the spinal column. Help your spinal column, and your nervous system will be grateful. A well-balanced system rests principally on these well-known basic elements:

- good-quality sleep;
- proper nutrition;
- adequate hydration;
- good emotional balance;
- effective breathing;
- satisfaction of needs;
- adequate physical exercise.

Let's take the example of the majority of North Americans these days: he sleeps six hours a night, he sleeps lightly, he eats processed foods and drinks coffee, he doesn't drink a lot of water, he took his last deep breath three years ago, he is going through a lot of stress at work and at home, and he hasn't trained for over a year. I'm sure you'll agree that chances are good that this person is feeling more than a little tension in his back!

Physical training helps expend energy — something that is entirely normal and natural for humans to do, and something they need as much as water and food.

On page 192, you will find exercises especially designed to rebalance the nervous system. At the same time, remember that any way to expend your energy is good for your body.

Are You Too Sympathetic?

The autonomic nervous system has two branches: the sympathetic and the parasympathetic nervous system. A balance between these two systems is necessary for the body to function properly. An imbalance can lead to different symptoms associated with a mode that is either too sympathetic, too parasympathetic, or a combination of both.

	SYMPATHETIC SYSTEM	PARASYMPATHETIC SYSTEM
Linked to...	Recovering energy	Expending energy
Location of nerves	In the skull and sacrum	Along the spinal column
Type of situation	"There's a fire. I have to dash out."	"I just ate. I have to digest."
Possible problems	• Tachycardia (rapid pulse) • Tendency to lose weight • Tendency to feel hot • Dry mouth • Dry skin	• Bradycardia (slow pulse) • Tendency to gain weight • Tendency to be cold • Excessive salivation • Clammy hands or feet

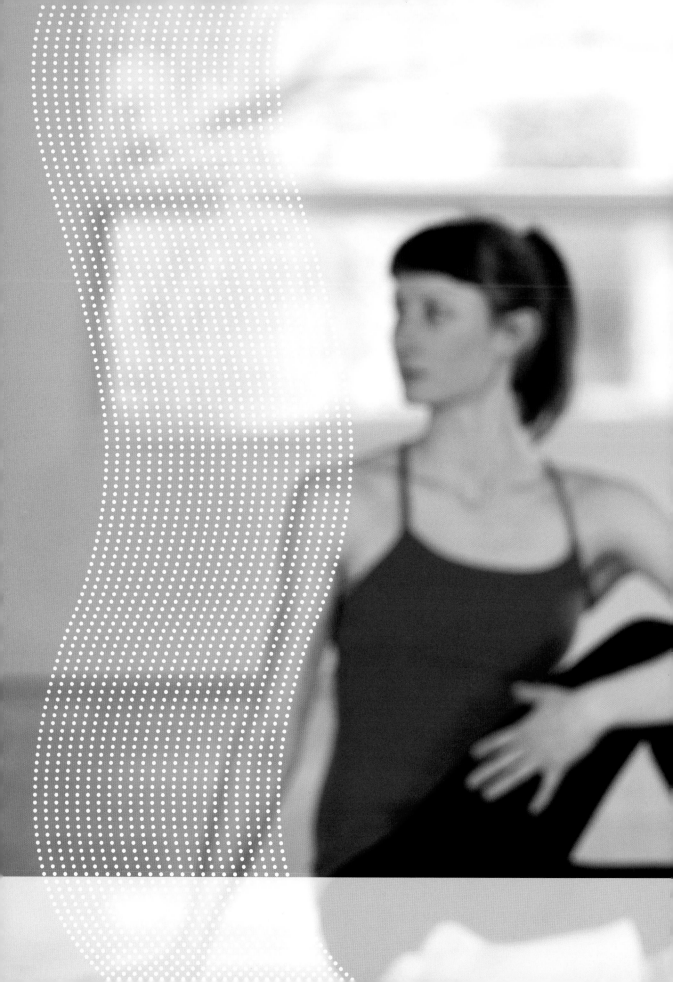

CHAPTER 5: THE PROGRAM

Overcoming Obstacles

It happens to most of us: you start an exercise program with the best of intentions, and a few weeks later, you realize you're nowhere near your goals. If you're reading this book, you're probably motivated to start applying the principles and doing the exercises you've learned. To increase your chances of success, it's best to first identify the three main reasons why people abandon an exercise program and then find ways to get around these obstacles.

1. Lack of Time

Not having time is the most common excuse for not training. It is more a case of not taking the time. We all have 15 minutes a day to devote to our health. All you need is a little goodwill and some strategy. Even if you have young children, even if you work long hours, you can find the time. Here are a few suggestions on how to make the most of your time:

- Spend 15 minutes less in front of the computer (You don't need to read the news one more time!).
- Spend 15 minutes less in front of the television.
- Do 15 minutes of exercises while watching television (it's better than nothing).
- Take 15 minutes to relax before going to bed (the bonus is that you will sleep better).

2. Fatigue

Are you one of those people who end the workday completely exhausted? If so, do you think this fatigue is really physical? Unless you are a professional cyclist, chances are that your fatigue is much more mental than physical. Mental fatigue is real. Anyone who has worked at a computer terminal for long hours can attest to this — after a day of work, the body and mind need to rest, but they also need to move. You can always sink into the sofa, but don't do it for too long. Are you tired? Move! After exercising, you will feel much more energetic than you did beforehand.

The hardest part is shaking off the lethargy that draws you like a magnet to the hollow space between the cushions. Have you ever attempted to get up from your armchair and found that you had no strength to move, but instead completely captivated by a mindless television show? Your brain is in passive mode and essentially functioning with non-revitalizing brain waves. Your mind and body are disconnected. This fatigue is not real, however. Your body is actually full of potential energy that is just begging to be liberated.

Reconnection Routine
This exercise routine will help you get your body and spirit working again.

1. Relaxation
Stand with your feet apart, aligned with your hips, and start by relaxing the following areas, one by one:

- the space between your eyes;
- your facial muscles;
- your jaw;
- your shoulders.

2. Reconnection With the Mind
Close your eyes and visualize an X.

3. Reconnection With Breathing
Breathe slowly, allowing your abdomen to expand, without effort.

4. Reconnection With the Central Axis
- Slowly contract your pelvic floor muscles.
- Contract your transversus abdominis muscle (belly muscle) and pull your navel inward.
- Push the tip of your tongue to the top of your skull.

5. Grounding
Visualize your feet spreading roots deep into the floor.

6. Elongation
Visualize a string attached to the top of your skull. With each inhalation, your spinal column lengthens and your skull is pulled upward effortlessly.

X = Focus

Do you want to improve your focus and concentration? Here's an exercise that comes from an educational kinesiology program called Brain Gym. Visualize an X, or even look at an X drawn on a sheet of paper. The action of visualizing an X calls on both hemispheres in the brain and requires good communication between them. I like to use this exercise with my students to help them with focused learning. Sometimes I include photos containing hidden X's in my visual presentations and ask them to find them. Use this guide as needed when studying or for concentrating your attention at an important moment.

Reconnecting can be done in just three minutes. At the beginning, it is normal to need more time, but with practice, you will soon manage to relax, focus your attention, breathe properly, ground yourself and adopt a good posture. Personally, I often do all of these steps at the same time, especially when I don't have much time (between two treatments, for example). Even writing this book required a few reconnecting sessions! One of my patients has become so efficient at the steps that he goes through them in the space of a breath (inhalation + exhalation).

3. Lack of Guidance

Once people have found the time and energy to train, they may still abandon their routine due to lack of guidance. Hiring a qualified personal trainer is often the best solution. A good trainer will motivate you and modify your program as needed. If you have back problems, make sure that your trainer is qualified on this subject.

If you train alone, you need to find ways to motivate yourself and to gauge your progress in relation to your objectives. See the guide, Chart 24 on page 249, a tool I use at my clinic and my training studio to guide patients.

Chart 24

This guide is based on a 24-day cycle. Why 24? The number corresponds to the number of vertebrae. It also represents an adequate period of time for observing results, and it goes by more quickly than a monthly plan. Photocopy the chart on page 249.

How to Use Chart 24

Every day, Chart 24 reminds you to devote a minimum amount of time to caring for your back by asking you the following questions:

- Did I exercise my back today?
- Did I remember to use my body effectively today?

On the chart, you will find an element that should be noted every day in your back-care resolutions. Even if you remembered just one of these elements once during the day, you can check off the box.

What Is the Condition of My Back?

It is a good idea to evaluate the general condition of your back. Use your posture and your level of energy to evaluate your condition on a scale of 1 to 10.

Examples:
- **1 out of 10** Posture completely collapsed and very little energy
- **5 out of 10** Good posture half the time with medium-level energy
- **10 out of 10** Excellent posture and full of energy

Here is how to fill out the chart:

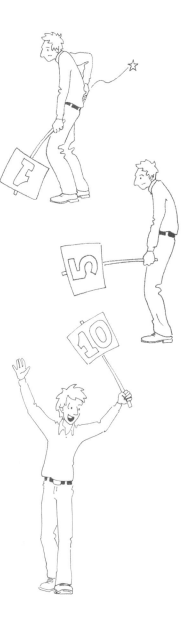

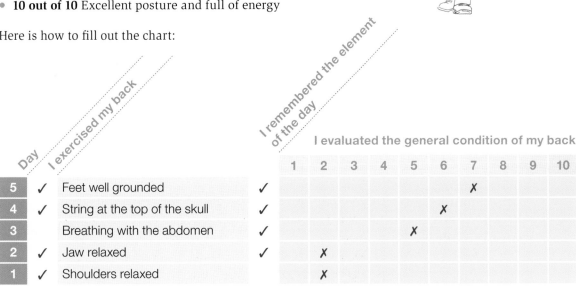

Day	I exercised my back		I remembered the element of the day	I evaluated the general condition of my back									
				1	2	3	4	5	6	7	8	9	10
5	✓	Feet well grounded	✓							X			
4	✓	String at the top of the skull	✓						X				
3		Breathing with the abdomen	✓					X					
2	✓	Jaw relaxed	✓		X								
1	✓	Shoulders relaxed			X								

Chart 24 is an excellent guide that is particularly useful in the early months of your program. After awhile, taking care of your back will be second nature to you. For a complete 24-day chart, see page 249.

Next Steps

After recommending back exercises to my patients, I have noticed when I see them a few weeks later that most of them have kept up their program and eventually their back problem is resolved. But this is when many of them stop caring about their back. Nevertheless, it is important to stick with the program, for two reasons:

- to be able to exercise the back with greater ease and without pain;
- to keep problems from recurring.

Continue your exercises and your back will understand that it can no longer play tricks on you.

Nine Tips for Succeeding in Your Program

Once the main obstacles are eliminated, here are nine ways to help you make an exercise program part of your daily routine.

1. Find the Right Moment

The people who exercise regularly have a time of day set aside for this activity. Any time is good as long as it works for you. Some prefer early mornings, starting their day with an exercise routine, while others do a series of stretches, like a sacred ritual, before going to bed.

In short, find the moment best suited to your needs, and come up with alternative solutions, just in case your plans change, for example, if you have a late night out.

Suggested Workout Times

Upon waking
During the morning break
During the midday break
During the afternoon break
After work
Before or after cardio training
While dinner is simmering on the stove
Upon returning from an evening walk
During the late news broadcast
Before going to bed

A few notes to consider when working out:

- When you first wake up in the morning, your body needs time to warm up sufficiently. Because your internal muscle temperature is at its lowest, the exercises must be done slowly — especially flexibility and strengthening exercises.
- After a meal, it is best to wait at least an hour before exercising. Strengthening exercises and cardio require that you wait more than 90 minutes. The body needs adequate time and a large blood supply in order to digest.
- Exercises done during breaks at work have the advantage of restoring energy and encouraging greater concentration and efficiency.

- Before going to bed, the best exercises are those targeting flexibility, breathing and balance. They encourage better sleep, and thus better recovery. Strengthening and cardio exercises tend to stimulate the body and delay sleep. It's up to you to see how you react. Some people do a complete one-hour routine consisting of lots of strengthening just before going to bed, and then sleep like babies.

2. Find the Right Place

Some people say they don't do their exercises because there isn't enough space in their home. If that's the case, for the sake of your back, find a solution. You only need a small space for most of the exercises.

Find a space that inspires you and rearrange it, if necessary. Doing your exercises on the cold floor of the kitchen with the whirring of the fridge beside you is perhaps not the most inspiring place.

At Home

- Find a room that can be free at the time when you do your exercises (away from your spouse and children). When you're ready to exercise, nothing should distract you.
- Distinguish the exercise period from the rest of the day. Diffuse the lighting, burn a candle, turn off the TV, put on music, take out your exercise mat — whatever you wish, as long as you get into a different mode.
- The equipment used (exercise mat, weights, elastic band, etc.) should be easily accessible in your room. A yoga mat rolls up easily and takes up little space.
- Your printed guide should be easily at hand. It's best to keep it somewhere in your exercise room.

At the Office

- Find a room (typically your office) or somewhere you can be alone during your break and leave your exercise mat there, hidden if necessary.
- If possible, go outside and find a quiet place such as a park.

In the Gym

- The area where the flexibility exercise mats are kept is usually a good place to stretch out.

3. Discover Your Back

To do your training program properly (like anything else), you should know what you're doing. If you're reading this book, you are probably learning a lot more about your back. This will make your training that much more effective.

4. Aim for Frequency

For all types of training, what has the most impact on results is not duration or intensity, but frequency. This is usually measured by the number of training sessions a week.

This rule applies to many activities. It is better to study often (even for a short period of time), than to study once for a long period of time. It is better to ride your bicycle for 1 hour 4 times a week than once a week for 4 hours. Some disciplined athletes train twice a day. This strategy can also be used when it comes to the back. I often do two short routines each day, one focusing on strengthening (earlier in the day) and the other on flexibility, mobility, breathing and restoring balance (at the end of the day). The idea is to do your exercises regularly, at least every other day (three to four times a week). If you manage to do them almost every day, you only need a short routine to obtain good results over the long term.

Four Examples of Effective Workout Routines

	Frequency	Training	Duration of training	Total duration for the week
1	3 to 4 times a week	Complete routine	30 to 60 minutes	1:30 to 4 hours
2	2 to 3 times a week + 2 to 3 times a week	Complete routine Short routine	30 to 60 minutes 5 to 15 minutes	1:10 to 3:45 hours
3	Once a week + 2 times a week + 2 times a week	Complete routine Medium routine Short routine	30 to 60 minutes 15 to 30 minutes 5 to 15 minutes	1:10 to 2:30 hours
4	5 to 6 times a week	Short routine	5 to 15 minutes	25 minutes to 1:30 hours

5. You Don't Need to Have Eternity Ahead of You

Some people get discouraged because their training session takes too long to complete. Going to the gym, for example, can take more than two hours when you factor in travel time, the training session and a shower. Keeping this up regularly is tough.

You will notice that it doesn't actually take a lot of time to care for your back. In the above table, the average time to complete a training session is just 15 minutes a day — up to 60 minutes for the most zealous. Even if you exercise just 5 minutes a day, with good, targeted exercises, you will have great results.

Some of my patients only do three flexibility exercises before going to bed, which take a maximum of three minutes, and they say that they still feel a big difference.

6. Take Holidays

For any type of activity, it's a good idea to take a break from time to time. Rest assured that your body will not deteriorate if you stop exercising for a few days. So don't feel guilty about taking holidays. It is even strongly recommended. After five days, however, the body does begin to lose its form.

Don't feel guilty, on the other hand, if you can't resist exercising. If that is the case, so much the better. However, I still encourage you to take a break, just so you can see how you feel.

After a break (especially a long one), you need to get your rhythm back. We have a tendency to quickly forget our routine. Make a note in your agenda or on your computer — whatever strategy works best — to remind you to get back to your good habits.

<table>
<tr><td colspan="3">Minimum Recommended Break</td></tr>
<tr><td>In a week</td><td>▶</td><td>One day</td></tr>
<tr><td>In a month</td><td>▶</td><td>Three consecutive days</td></tr>
<tr><td>In a year</td><td>▶</td><td>At least a week</td></tr>
</table>

7. Use a Minimum Amount of Equipment

Exercise equipment (muscle-building apparatus, cardio devices, weights) can be useful but won't be if you're exercising outside. To be autonomous, you shouldn't depend on equipment.

8. Think "Specific Training"

Specific training is linked directly to the targeted goal, while general training is not. For example, if your goal is to run 3 miles (5 km) in a marathon this autumn, your specific training will involve running at an intense level that closely resembles the speed in the competitive event. You can swim, cycle, or even practice your lawn bowling — all of them are good for fitness, but they will not train you in a specific fashion to reach your goal. These activities fit into the category of general training, in this case.

Spinal Training Tip

The Spinal Training method does not require any equipment. So it can follow you wherever you go!

9. Pleasure Most of All

Like any activity you're doing in the long term, getting pleasure from it is essential. Here are some examples of the pleasure that comes from Spinal Training:

Spinal Training Tip

If you want to see good results for your back, you need to do specific exercises. Spinal Training works exactly in this way.

- the pleasure of having better posture, without effort;
- the pleasure of no longer feeling back pain;
- the pleasure of feeling in control of a situation;
- the pleasure of understanding how the back works;
- the pleasure of feeling satisfied after a good workout;
- the pleasure of reconnecting with one's breathing;
- the pleasure of feeling firm and strong:
- the pleasure of feeling energized and relaxed at the same time.

This non-exhaustive list is based on the comments I usually hear in my training studio after a session. Even if you experience just one of these pleasures, it's worth putting some effort into your training. In scientific terms, the pleasure that comes from exercising is due to a significant secretion of hormones, including endorphins and dopamine. These natural drugs released by the body have a powerful influence over your body and mind. Take advantage of them — they're free and legal!

Quick Back Self-Assessment

This self-assessment for your back will really help you understand your back's specific needs and help you determine which training will be the most beneficial. Identifying your strengths and weaknesses will help you select the routines that best suit your situation. It will also help you measure your progress in a tangible way.

"Flex" and "Power" Self-Assessment

To determine whether you are the "flex" type (good flexibility), the "power" type (good muscle strength), or balanced (a combination of both), do the following tests, tabulate your scores for "flex" and "power" exercises and then compare your results at the end of this chapter.

Flexibility ("Flex")
Flexibility of the Hamstring Muscles

With your heels against the wall and your feet aligned with your hips, using a ruler or sheet of paper between your legs, lean forward as far as possible (go slowly, and stop if you feel pain).

Your fingertips are...

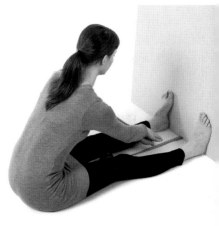

	Woman*	Man
more than 12 in (30 cm) from the wall	1	2
6 to 12 in (15 to 30 cm) from the wall	4	6
2 to 6 in (5 to 15 cm) from the wall	7	9
0 to 2 in (0 to 5 cm) from the wall	10	11
touching the wall	12	12

Flexibility of Large Dorsal Muscle

Assume the following position and lean as far as you can to one side (see Exercise 13 on page 122).

For you, this exercise is...

	Woman*	Man
A difficult; uncomfortable	1	2
B fairly easy	4	5
C easy; wide range of movement	8	8

* Women are naturally more flexible than men, which explains the difference in the scoring.

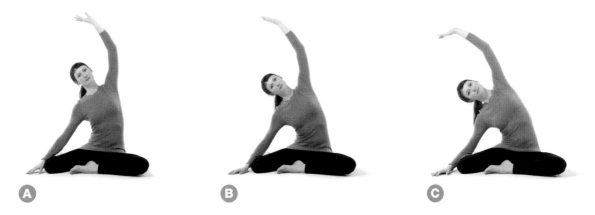

A   B   C

Muscle Strength ("Power")

(see Exercise 65 on page 185)

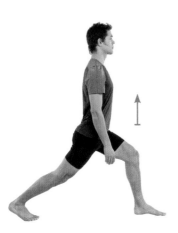

Squat

With your feet spread wide apart front and back and your back straight, do 10 lunges, descending until your front thigh is parallel to the ground. Alternate legs.

For you, this exercise is...

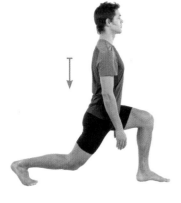

too difficult; impossible to do 10 repetitions	1
difficult; requires effort	4
moderately easy; it would have been possible to do more	7
easy; requires little effort	10

Plank

(see Exercise 62 on page 182)
Assume this position, with your back straight, and hold it for a maximum of 1 minute. Stop if you feel pain.

You managed to hold the position...

less than 10 seconds; this exercise is too difficult	1
10 to 20 seconds	4
20 to 40 seconds	7
more than 40 seconds	10

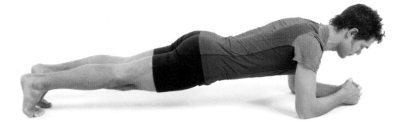

Results

Once you tabulate your "flex" and "power" scores, calculate the difference between the two scores.

	"Flex"	Balanced	"Power"
Difference in results	10 points more in "flex"	Less than 10 points difference between "power" and "flex"	10 points more in "power"
Conclusion (see page 209)	You need to focus on strengthening exercises. Do Power routine P1, P2 and P3	You need balance training. Do Spinal routine S1, S2 and S3	You need to focus on flexibility exercises. Do Flex routine F1, F2 and F3

Complete Self-Assessment

If you want to have a better idea of the general condition of your back, do the following tests, which will only take a few minutes longer. Naturally, I suggest that you work with a qualified trainer, who can assess you fully and then give you advice on developing your routine.

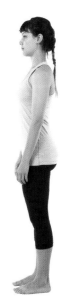

Relaxation

In the standing position, which one of these statements applies to you?

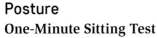

My jaw muscles are...	very tense	1	*My shoulders are...*	very tense	1
	tense	3		tense	3
	slightly tense	5		slightly tense	5
	completely relaxed	7		completely relaxed	7.5

Posture
One-Minute Sitting Test

Remain in a seated position for 1 minute with your back very straight.

For you, this exercise is...

very difficult; impossible to sit up straight	1
difficult; requires effort	3
fairly easy; requires slight effort	7
very easy; no effort required	10

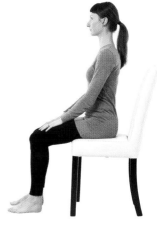

Test for Balancing on One Leg

Assume this position and try to hold it for 1 minute. (Because balance will vary from one side to the other, try doing it on the other side, too, and taking an average score.)

You manage to...

hold this position with difficulty, putting the foot down several times during the minute	1
hold this position for a maximum of 20 seconds at a time	3
hold this position for 21 to 45 seconds	6
hold this position for 46 to 60 seconds	9
hold this position easily for 1 minute or even longer	10

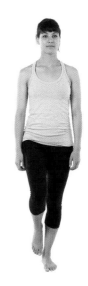

Mobility

Test for Rotating the Back While Seated

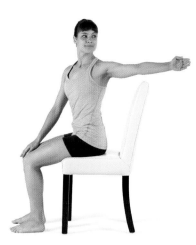

Sit facing forward with both feet on the ground, raise one arm to the side until it is parallel to the ground, then rotate backward as far as possible while turning your head and trunk. Stop before you feel any discomfort. Alternate sides and calculate your score according to the average.

You rotate your arm...

less than 30° toward the back	1
between 30 and 60° toward the back	4
more than 60° toward the back	8

Test for Tilting the Back While Standing

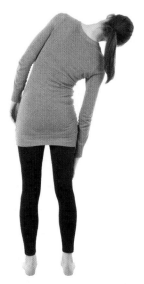

While standing and facing forward, slide your arm sideways down the length of your leg, as far as you can go. Stop before you feel any discomfort.

The fingertips reach...

higher than ⅔ of the thigh	1
between ⅔ of the thigh and the knee	3
to the knee	5
below the knee	7

Breathing

Abdominal Breathing

Lying on your back, breathe and let your abdomen expand, without effort, for five inhalations and exhalations.

Which one of these statements applies to you?

it's impossible	1
it's difficult	3
my abdomen expands a little, without too much effort	6
my abdomen expands a lot, with no effort	10

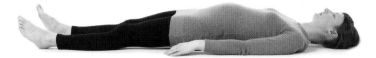

Interpreting the Results

Overall Score

In the following table you can fill in the scores you got on each test from pages 97 to 100. Add them up for a total score out of 100. You can always redo this self-assessment to measure your progress.

Weaknesses to Target

You will also find scores that indicate weakness in a given element. Lower scores mean you should focus more on these elements to improve the condition of your back.

	Flexibility	Muscle strength	Relaxation	Posture	Mobility	Breathing	Total
My results	/20	/20	/15	/20	/15	/10	/100
To work on if I scored:	11 points or less ☐	8 points or less ☐	6 points or less ☐	10 points or less ☐	6 points or less ☐	4 points or less ☐	

Notes : _____

_____

_____

_____

_____

_____

_____

_____

_____

_____

_____

_____

_____

_____

_____

_____

_____

_____

_____

_____

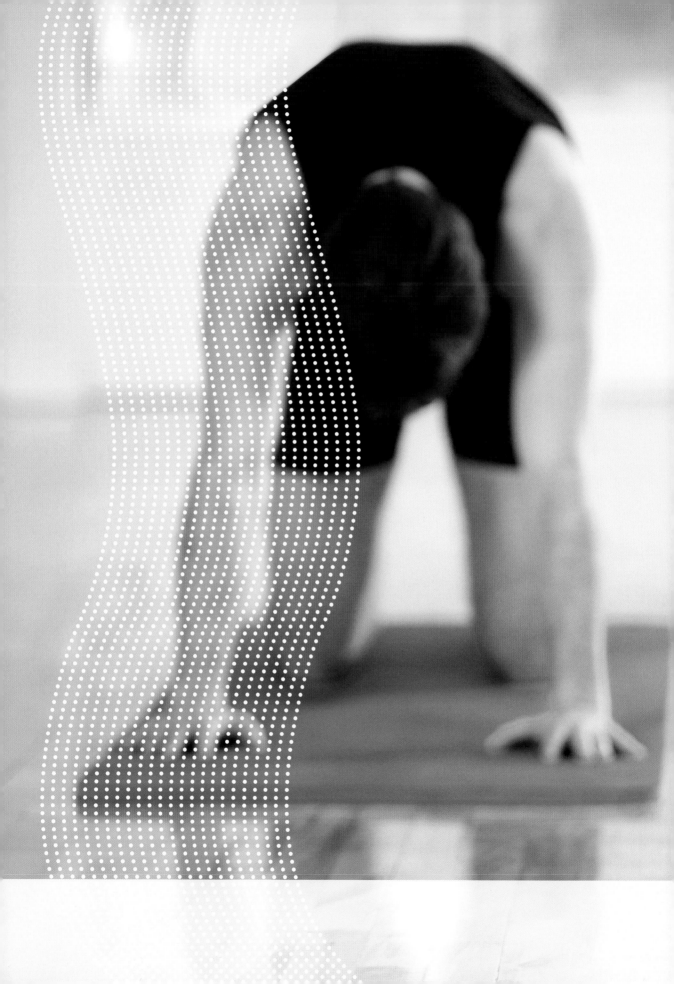

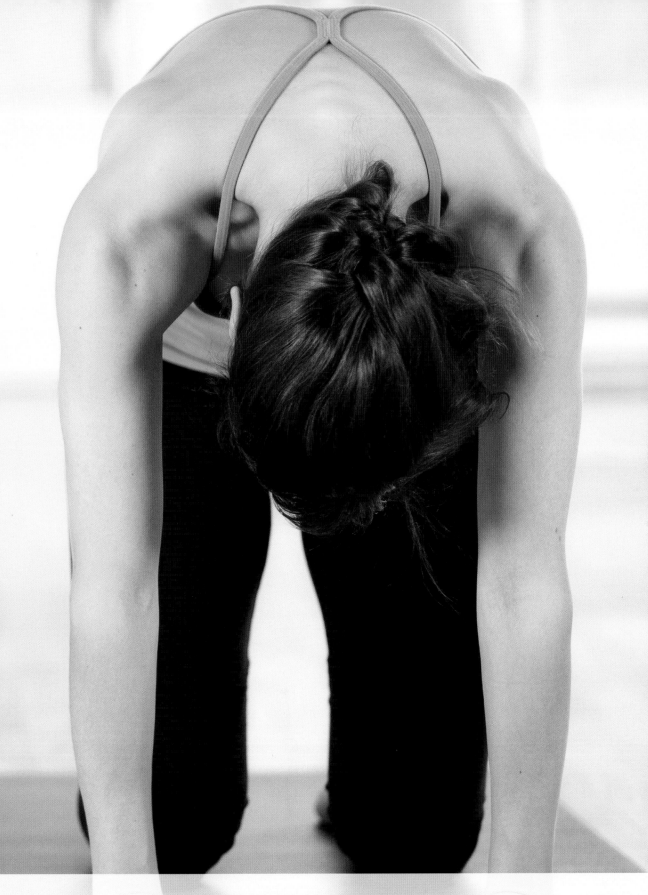

CHAPTER 6: EXERCISES

On the Road to Good Health

It's time to get your back moving. The following exercises will help you stretch, mobilize, strengthen and revitalize the back. With 80 exercises to choose from, you'll find more than enough postures to meet your back's needs. Think of these exercises as individual recipes that will eventually be combined to create a robust menu. Keep in mind that just one exercise, done regularly, can make a big difference in the health of your back.

List of Exercises

Basics

1 Elongation of the Spinal Column
2 Grounding
3 Grounding and Elongation
4 Contraction of the Transversus Abdominis
5 Contraction of the Pelvic Floor
6 Contraction of the Transversus Abdominis and Pelvic Floor

Flexibility

7 Hamstring Stretch (Standing)
8 Hamstring Stretch (Lying Down)
9 Calf Stretch
10 Deep Gluteal Stretch (with Pelvic Floor Stretch)
11 Iliopsoas Stretch
12 Quadriceps Stretch
13 Large Dorsal and Quadratus Lumborum Stretch
14 Quadratus Femoris Stretch
15 Lumbar Spinal Stretch
16 Lumbar Spinal Stretch (Squatting)
17 Lumbar Spinal Stretch (Lying Down)
18 Posterolateral Chain Stretch
19 Pectoral (Major/Minor) Stretch
20 Cervical Spinal Stretch
21 Levator Scapulae and Upper Trapezius Stretch
22 Elongation of Lower Back

Mobility

23 Cat/Cow Pose
24 Cat/Cow Pose (Alternative)
25 Tail Wag
26 Cat Stretch
27 Back Twist
28 Back Twist (Advanced)
29 Pelvic Tilt
30 Prune Face/Baby Lion Face
31 Relaxation of the Suboccipital Muscles
32 Neck Figure 8's
33 Windshield Wipers
34 The X
35 Reach for the Sky

Breathing

36 Release
37 Abdominal and Sternal Breathing
38 Deep Exhalation
39 Rebalancing Breathing
40 Child's Pose
41 Pumping Abdominal Twist
42 Relaxation of Diaphragm

Posture

43 Bounces
44 Stimulating the Deep Muscles of the Back
45 Balancing on One Leg
46 Dorsal Muscle Elongation
47 Helical Elongation of the Back
48 Helical Elongation of the Neck
49 Helical Elongation of the Lumbar Muscles
50 Helical Elongation with Lunge
51 Helical Elongation on One Leg
52 Helical Elongation with Limb Spirals
53 Relaxation of the Lateral Muscles
54 Rhythmic Neck Rotation
55 Slump/Straighten Up
56 Compression/Elongation

Strengthening

57 Half Bridge
58 Single-Leg Half Bridge
59 Leg Circles
60 Balancing Table
61 Balancing Table with Diagonals
62 Plank (or Half Plank)
63 Side Plank (or Half Side Plank)
64 Rotary Plank on Wall
65 Lunge
66 Diagonal
67 Squat/Elongation
68 Half Roll-Up
69 Oblique Half Roll-Up
70 Ultimate Pelvic Floor Contraction
71 Pelvic Balancing

Cardio

Refer to the section dealing with cardio, page 82.

Balance

72 Overall Balance
73 Sleeping Car
74 Central Axis
75 Back-Relief Position
76 Express Temple and Neck Relaxation
77 Shoulders and Neck Relaxation
78 Chest, Shoulders and Neck Relaxation
79 Overall Back Relaxation
80 Neuromuscular Relaxation

Basics

These exercises are designed to familiarize you with the fundamentals of the Spinal Training method — the principles of elongation and grounding, as well as the activation of the core and deep muscles of the spinal column. It is essential to master these basics before you do the rest of the exercises in this book.

The Key To Succeed

It is important to fully understand the exercises before doing them. Give yourself time to master them.

Duration

The duration of each exercise varies. Work on the quality of the movement, taking more time than recommended, if needed.

Caution

The exercises should not be accompanied by back pain (during or after).

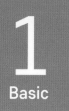

Elongation of the spinal column
▶ for all

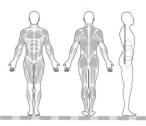

One of the basic principles in activating the deep muscles of the central axis and developing good posture, elongation of the spinal column is the first exercise to master. It is the keystone of postural exercise and should be applied to all of the exercises as well as in daily life.

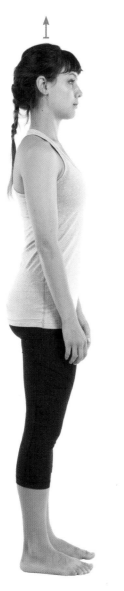

Initial Position

Standing, the feet aligned with the hips.

Action

As you inhale, pull the top of your skull upward and the tip of your coccyx (tailbone) downward. As you exhale, imagine that the forces pulling you are disappearing and that your spinal column is resuming its original length.

Once you have mastered elongation, practice holding it for longer periods of time, and always without straining.

Visualization

Imagine that a small string attached to the top of your skull is slowly pulling your head upward. Your head should remain in the neutral position, without bending or stretching.

You can also imagine that your head is a hot-air balloon and your pelvis is the basket. Your spinal column is suspended under the balloon.

The Key To Succeed

Do this exercise with a minimum amount of effort.

AVOID

▶ Letting your spinal column sag
▶ Tensing your back muscles

EFFECTS

▶ Better posture
▶ More efficient breathing
▶ Back pain relief

DURATION

▶ 1 to 2 minutes or 5 to 10 breaths

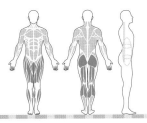
Although it is recommended to hold your head high, you still need to keep your feet firmly on the ground. By grounding yourself, you help the Earth's gravitational forces assist with your posture and movement, and help you maintain your balance. In Chinese medicine, it is said that we tap into Earth's energy through the soles of our feet. Grounding activates the proprioceptors in the feet in an optimal way.

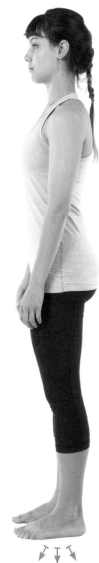

Initial Position

Standing, the feet (ideally barefoot) and aligned with the hips opened up naturally (at a 20- to 30-degree angle).

Action

Be aware of your feet in contact with the floor and the gravitational force that is pulling you toward the center of the Earth. Take note of your footprints on the floor before and after the exercise to see if there is a difference.

Visualization

Imagine you are a tree. Picture roots growing out of your toes, heels and other areas of your soles. Let these roots grow deep into the floor. This visualization will usually give you greater stability and better balance.

You can also imagine that your feet are attached to the floor by suction cups.

The Key To Succeed

Clearly visualize your feet in contact with the floor.

AVOID	EFFECTS	DURATION
▸ Putting more weight on one leg than the other	▸ Better posture ▸ Increased proprioception ▸ More energy	▸ 1 to 2 minutes or 5 to 10 breaths

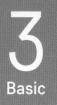

3

Basic

Grounding and elongation
▶ for all

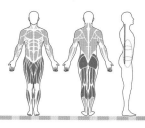

With your head held high and your feet firmly planted, you're reaching the best of both worlds. It is a basic exercise that can be done any time or place. Grounding is an excellent way to get centered and reacquainted with your body, and it only takes 2 minutes. You can do the active moving or passive static version as you wish. Try them with your eyes closed to make it more challenging. Both versions are effective. You can alternate or choose your favorite one.

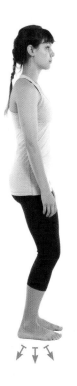 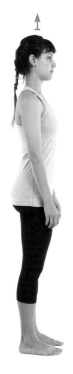

Moving Version
Initial Position

Standing, the feet aligned with the hips.

Action

As you exhale, slowly bend your knees and put more weight on your feet to help them be grounded. As you inhale, lengthen your legs and spinal column, imagining that a string attached to the top of your skull is pulling your entire body upward.

Static Version
Action

Start by planting your feet firmly on the floor. Then, lengthen your spinal column so that you are elongating and grounding yourself at the same time.

AVOID

▶ Bending your knees too much while planting your feet

EFFECTS

▶ Better posture
▶ More efficient breathing
▶ Back pain relief
▶ Greater energy

DURATION

▶ 1 to 2 minutes or 5 to 10 breaths

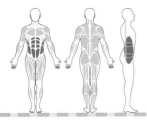

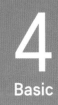

Mastering the contraction of the transversus abdominis muscle is essential to activating the core muscles. The transversus abdominis is a veritable lumbar support belt. It works with the oblique muscles to stabilize the core muscles and initiate movement. This movement can be practiced lying down, sitting or standing, at home, in the car or at the computer. You just have to remember to do it. Over time, as you initiate this movement with your core muscles, contracting your transversus abdominis will come naturally.

Some people have difficulty contracting the transversus abdominis and need more practice to master it. If this is the case with you, persevere, and your back will be grateful.

Initial Position
Lying on the back.

Action
As you exhale, pull in your navel toward your spinal column. As you inhale, allow your abdomen to expand.

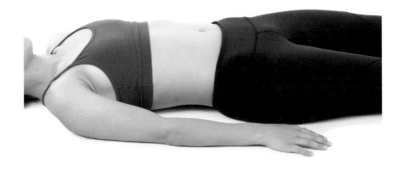

Visualization
1. Imagine you are pulling up a zipper, between your pubic bone and navel, on a pair of pants that are too tight.
2. Imagine you are stepping into a freezing-cold swimming pool (the second the water reaches your pubic bone, you pull in your navel to protect your internal organs).
3. Lying on your back, place your hands on your lower abdomen and cough, which should trigger a strong reflex contraction in your abdomen.

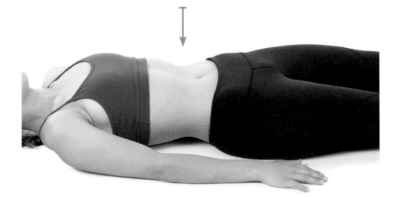

AVOID	EFFECTS	DURATION
▸ Tipping your pelvis ▸ Bending your trunk	▸ Greater control of the core muscles ▸ Greater stability ▸ More efficient breathing	▸ 10 to 20 repetitions

5

Basic

Contraction of the pelvic floor

▶ for all

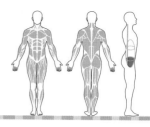

Contracting the pelvic floor muscles is essential to helping the back function properly. It should be a part of any exercise you do. For men, it is the best exercise for the prostate and should be done on a regular basis. It is also an important exercise for women, especially in the case of a descended bladder, and before or after childbirth. In any case, it is a basic exercise everyone should master. The center of the pelvic floor in women is located between the vagina and anus, and in men it is between the scrotum and anus.

Initial Position

Lying on the back, sitting or standing.

Action

As you exhale, contract your pelvic floor muscles. As you inhale, relax them.

Visualization

Contract your pelvic floor muscles by pulling in your abdomen. Take care not to needlessly contract your superficial gluteal muscles (the gluteus maximus, for example). The muscle work in this exercise is both deep and subtle.

The Key To Succeed

The ability to relax the muscles is as important as the ability to contract them.

Tip

You can also feel a contraction by tightening your urinary or anal sphincter. Don't focus too much on the sphincter muscles — if you exercise them too much, you may inadvertently modify their natural reflex. Bladder retention exercises should be avoided.

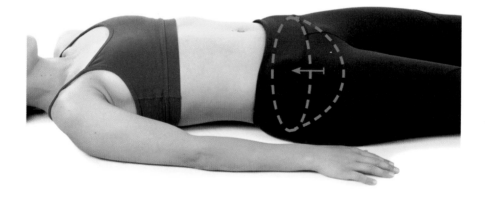

AVOID

▶ Contracting by using all of your gluteal muscles

EFFECTS

▶ Greater control of the core muscles
▶ Greater stability
▶ More efficient breathing

DURATION

▶ 10 to 20 repetitions

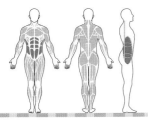
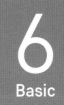
Once you master contracting the transversus abdominis and the pelvic floor separately, you can work on contracting both simultaneously. This contraction is totally natural because the muscles normally work as a team. The pelvic floor, transversus abdominis and oblique muscles (which also work during these exercises) are an essential part of the body's core muscles.

This exercise can be practiced in a variety of positions. You can train and reactivate your core muscles just about anywhere, while standing, sitting or lying down.

Initial Position
Lying on the back, sitting or standing.

Action
As you exhale, simultaneously contract your pelvic floor (pulling in your abdomen) and your transversus abdominis muscle (pulling in your navel toward your spinal column). As you inhale, relax your muscles, allowing your abdomen to expand.

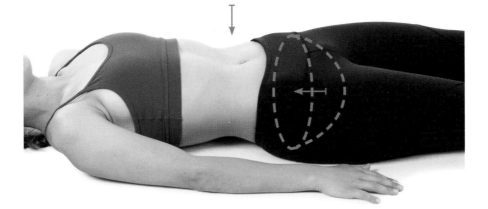

AVOID	EFFECTS	DURATION
▸ Putting the emphasis on contracting and forgetting to fully relax your muscles	▸ Greater control of the core muscles ▸ Greater stability ▸ More efficient breathing	▸ 10 to 20 repetitions

Flexibility

Flexibility exercises are also called stretches. They should target the muscles that have a tendency to be tense, since these cause imbalance that affect your back and posture. To help the tissues stretch more easily, these exercises should be done when your muscles and joints have been sufficiently warmed up.

The Keys To Succeed

Because body temperature is at its lowest upon awakening and gradually rises to its maximum by 6 p.m., morning is not typically the best time for stretching. It is better to awaken your body with mobility exercises (shown in the next section).

It is important to be able to hold a big stretch — about 90 to 95% of the maximum — while relaxing. It does no good to strain or to tense up while stretching. You will see the best results when you are capable of relaxing and breathing properly. Assume the stretching position slowly and gradually, and then hold it.

Duration

The stretch should be maintained for at least 30 seconds. Otherwise there will only be minimal improvement in suppleness. For better results, it is recommended that you hold the position for 45 seconds. For the best results, do each stretch twice. You can do a complete series and then start over again, or stretch on both sides and then start over again.

Caution

A stretch should not be accompanied by pain during or after the exercise. It should never be accompanied by numbness. You should never shake or jerk while stretching.

Hamstring stretch (standing)

▸ for all

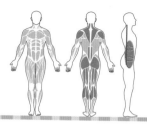

If you had to choose only one stretching exercise, the hamstring stretch would be the biggest contender. This version is practical because you can do it anywhere. It has the added advantage of improving balance and elongating the back, making it a very useful exercise for posture. The main challenge is to keep the back straight.

Initial Position

Standing, one foot on a raised surface like a chair.

Action

Pull your toes toward you, extend the palms of your hands toward the ceiling and then lean your trunk forward, keeping your back straight and arms extended, until you feel a slight pull on your hamstring.

If the exercise is too difficult, you can bend your knees slightly to help you be more flexible. You can also do the exercise with your arms down and at your sides.

The Key To Succeed

Keep your back straight and your spinal column elongated throughout the exercise.

The pulling sensation is often more intense in the calves than in the back of the thighs. This is entirely normal. In this exercise, we stretch the posterior chain, which includes the hamstrings and calves. The link in the chain that is normally the most tense is the one in which we feel the strongest pull.

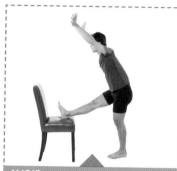

AVOID

▸ Rounding your back

EFFECTS

▸ Increased suppleness in the hamstring muscles
▸ Better posture
▸ Back pain relief

DURATION

▸ 45 seconds on each side

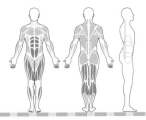

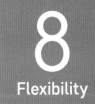

This unconventional stretch helps to disengage the hamstrings as well as relax the back. If you experience numbness in the legs and feet, bend your knee until it disappears.

Initial Position

Lying on the back, knees slightly bent (with a towel or elastic band under the toes of the leg to be stretched, for beginners).

Action

Bring your leg toward you, keeping it as straight as possible. Extend your heel toward the ceiling, flexing your toes toward the floor and pushing your knee away from your chest.

The Key To Succeed

The challenge is to keep your thigh from coming toward your chest while forcing your thigh and abdominal muscles to help you stretch the muscles in the back of your thigh.

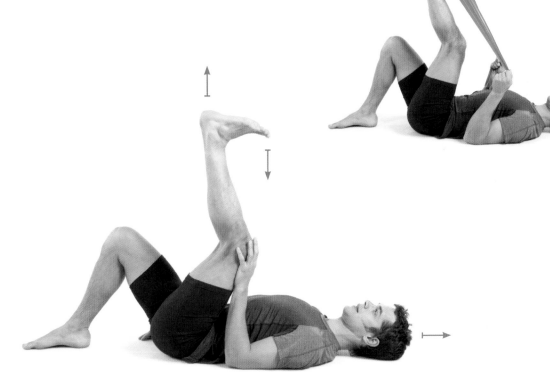

AVOID	EFFECTS	DURATION
▸ Moving your thigh away from your hand	▸ Increased suppleness in the hamstring muscles ▸ Better posture ▸ Back pain relief	▸ 45 seconds on each side

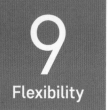
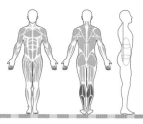
As part of the posterior chain that includes the back of the thighs and the muscles along the spinal column, the calves are often tense. High-heeled shoes are their worst enemy. The calves have a major impact on standing posture and need to be stretched. In this exercise, gastrocnemius muscles (medial and lateral heads) in the upper calf and the soleus muscles in the lower calf are stretched specifically for better results.

If you only have time for one stretch, work on the gastrocnemius muscle stretch. If you have more time or want to improve your suppleness, you should do the soleus muscle stretch as well.

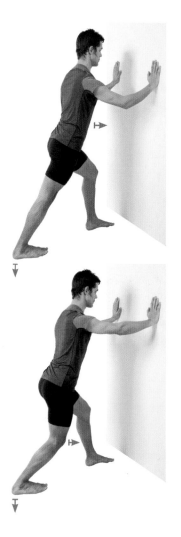

Gastrocnemius Muscles
Initial Position
Standing facing a wall, with one foot far behind the other. The hands are pressed against the wall at shoulder height. Arms are straight.

Action
Press the heel of your back leg into the floor and move your pelvis forward until you feel a pull in your hamstring, keeping the heel flat on the floor.

Soleus Muscle
Initial Position
Standing facing a wall, with on foot far behind the other and the knee slightly bent. The hands are pressed against the wall at shoulder height. Arms are straight.

Action
Move your pelvis forward, keeping the heel of your back leg flat on the floor and your knee bent.

Alternatives
Medial head: With the foot of your back leg turned inward 20 degrees, force your inside arch into the floor. Your heel must always be flat on the floor.
Lateral head: With the foot of your back leg turned outward 20 degrees, force your outer arch into the floor. Your heel must always be flat on the floor.

AVOID
▶ Lifting your heel off the floor
▶ Placing your feet too close together

EFFECTS
▶ Increased suppleness in the calves
▶ Better posture
▶ Back pain relief

DURATION
▶ 45 seconds on each side

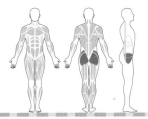
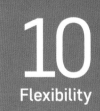
This exercise is very effective for releasing tension deeply entrenched in the buttock, which often comes from tension in the piriformis muscle. The trick is to stretch the deep gluteal muscles in a pumping motion while contracting the pelvic floor. I developed this exercise to release recurring tension in one of my patients and it has since helped many people.

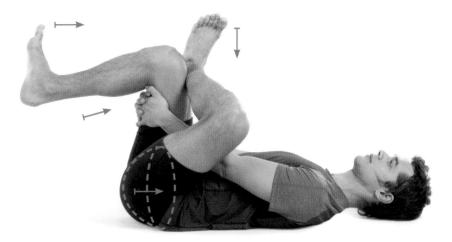

Initial Position
(For the Left Side)

Lying on the back, the left leg crossed and placed in front of the bent knee on the right leg.

Action

With your fingers laced behind your right thigh, pull your thigh toward your abdomen, then bring your toes (especially the little toe) toward your knees.

Once you feel a stretch in your gluteal muscles, inhale and contract your pelvic floor, then relax it as you exhale (pumping). Do the same on the right side.

The Key To Succeed

Really feel the stretch before pumping.

Tip

If you feel a sharp pain in your buttock, do this exercise very slowly, first stretching your buttock on the side where it doesn't hurt. Stretch without going all the way and without pumping. After stretching, if it feels better, try the exercise again and only pump lightly.

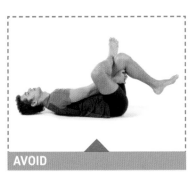

AVOID

▸ Extending your neck (use a cushion if needed to avoid)

EFFECTS

▸ Increased suppleness in the deep gluteal muscles
▸ Release tension in the pelvis
▸ Relief from sciatic nerve irritation

DURATION

▸ 5 pumps on each side (for about 45 seconds)

Iliopsoas stretch
▶ beginner to advanced

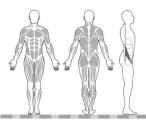

Because of our lifestyle, which often requires us to sit, our iliopsoas muscles often end up in a shortened position and need to be stretched. Start off slowly — for some people, stretching these muscles produces tension in the lower back. This exercise is recommended for people who work sitting down, as well as cyclists, runners, rowers and cross-country skiers.

It is important to do this stretch very slowly during the first attempts. Make sure you have mastered it before going further.

Beginner

Initial Position

Kneeling on one knee, with a chair or other stable object on one side for support. The forward foot should be aligned with the hips, and the back knee should be as far back as possible, slightly turned inward. For greater comfort, a cushion can be placed under the back knee.

Action

Move your pelvis forward (keeping your back straight) until you feel a full stretch in the front of the hip of your back leg. Extend the top of your head toward the ceiling.

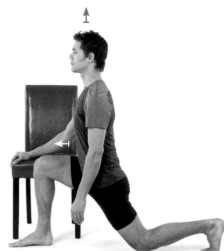

Advanced

Action

Without using a support, push your heel on your back leg backward while raising your knee, keep your pelvis low and contract your gluteal muscles.

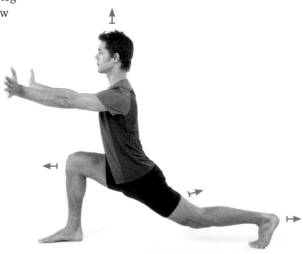

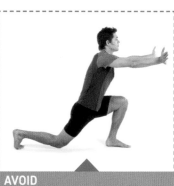

AVOID

▶ Rounding your back
▶ Leaning forward
▶ Keeping your legs too close together

EFFECTS

▶ Increased suppleness in the iliopsoas
▶ Back pain relief

DURATION

▶ 30 to 45 seconds on each side

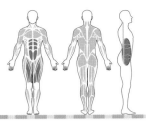
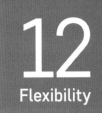
Some of the muscles in the front of the thighs (the right interior of the quadriceps) have a tendency to tense up. This stretch helps to relax them and improve your balance and posture. This exercise is ideally combined with the hamstring stretch (see Exercise 7 or 8). It is especially recommended for people who walk a lot as well as athletes.

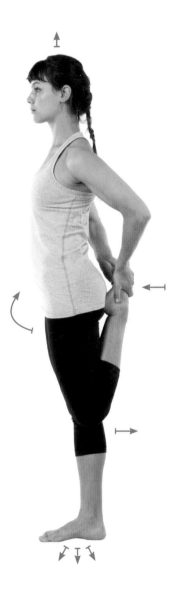

Initial Position
Standing, bend your leg back to touch your buttock (if possible) and hold the ankle or foot with both hands.

Action
1. Bring your heel toward your buttock.
2. Bring your knee back (while continuing the action in Step 1).
3. Bring your pubic bone toward your navel (while continuing the action in Steps 1 and 2). Maintain this position while elongating your spinal column.

Visualization
Imagine that a small string attached to the top of your skull is slowly pulling your head upward. At the same time, visualize that your foot is deeply rooted in the ground.

    Repeat the exercise with the other leg.

The Key To Succeed
Keep your spinal column elongated and stay firmly grounded.

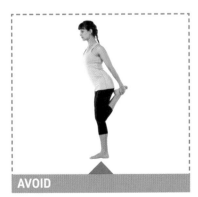

AVOID	EFFECTS	DURATION
▸ Bending your back forward ▸ Letting your heel move away from your buttock	▸ Increased suppleness in the thighs ▸ Increased proprioception ▸ Better posture	▸ 45 seconds on each side

13
Flexibility

Large dorsal and quadratus lumborum stretch
▶ for all

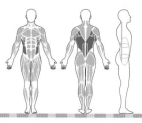

The large dorsal muscles of the back often display asymmetrical tension. Stretching them helps to correct this imbalance. This exercise stretches all of the lateral part of the chest and some of the quadratus lumborum, which is another muscle that tends to be tense. It is also a very good breathing exercise.

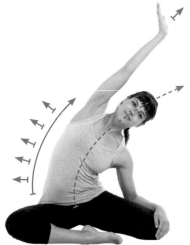

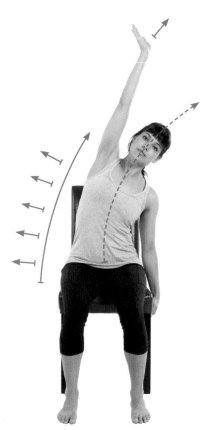

Stretch

Initial Position (For the Right Side)
Sitting, right leg folded in, foot close to the body. The left leg is behind, knee bent, heel close to the buttock.

Action
Extend the palm of your right hand toward the ceiling and lean to the left, keeping your spinal column elongated and your head extended in the same direction. Repeat the exercise on the opposite side.

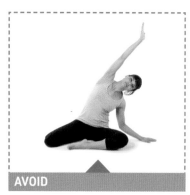

Alternate Position
People with knee or hip problems can do this exercise sitting on a chair.

The Key To Succeed
Breath to open up the side being stretched.

AVOID	EFFECTS	DURATION
▶ Leaning to the wrong side	▶ Increased lateral suppleness in the back	▶ 45 seconds on each side
▶ Losing length in the spinal column	▶ More efficient breathing	
	▶ Back pain relief	

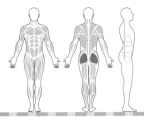

Inspired by the pigeon pose well known to those who do yoga postures, this exercise stretches quadratus femoris and the deep gluteal muscles. The little-known quadratus femoris is often tense, especially in people whose legs are naturally positioned far apart. Some people do not feel the stretch, and if that is the case, you can count yourself lucky! For the rest of us, this stretch is very effective in relaxing the hips and pelvis.

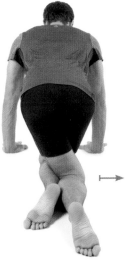

Initial Position (For the Right Side)

Starting on all fours, the left knee is crossed to the right behind the right knee, before the left leg is extended.

Action

Extend your left leg crossed over the right and sit on your right buttock. Then extend the left leg out behind you and bring your chest down as far as you can without discomfort. Repeat the exercise on the opposite side.

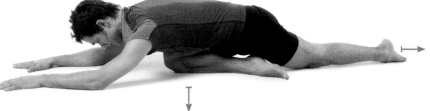

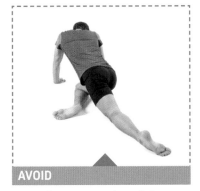

AVOID	**EFFECTS**	**DURATION**
▸ Putting too much weight on your hip	▸ Better posture ▸ More efficient breathing ▸ Back pain relief	▸ 45 seconds on each side

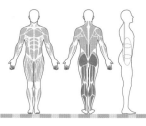

Tense lumbar spinal muscles prevent your abdominal muscles from functioning well, which is why they need to be stretched before you do abdominal exercises. They are often more tense on one side than the other. In this case, the unilateral version of this exercise is recommended. The ideal combination is a trio of stretches (unilateral on both sides, then bilateral).

In most people, the pulling sensation is strongest behind the thighs, which is normal because muscles here are typically tight.

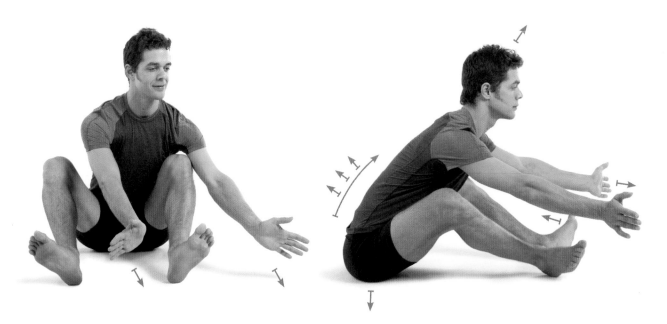

Unilateral Version

Initial Position
Sitting, both buttocks flat on the floor, knees bent.

Action (For the Right Side)
Push your hands forward and to the left at an approximately 30-degree seated angle.
  Repeat the exercise, pushing to the right.

Bilateral Version

Action
Push your hands forward and bring your fingers back, then expand your lower back as you inhale.

AVOID	EFFECTS	DURATION
▶ Extending your neck	▶ Increased suppleness in the lower back and back of the thighs ▶ Back pain relief	▶ 45 seconds on each side

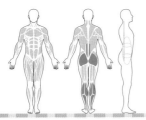
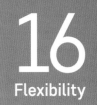
This position is assumed by people in a variety of different cultures when they're taking a break or just chatting with friends. It is not an easy position for everyone to hold, however, and anyone with fragile knees should abstain or proceed cautiously. An excellent exercise for unblocking the lower back, it requires a lot of flexibility in the calves and lower back as well as good mobility in the hips and pelvis. If you are comfortable in this position, try the alternate version, which encourages deeper breathing for a better workout.

This exercise is not recommended if you have knee problems or pain in your knee, hip or ankle. You should not attempt this exercise if you have a herniated disk.

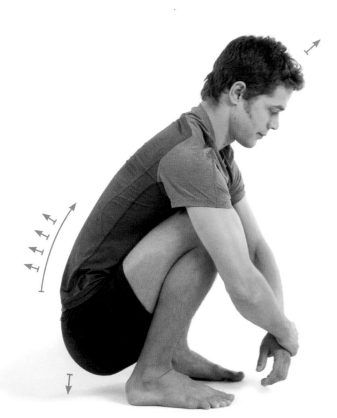

Initial Position
Crouching, the feet positioned wider than the hips. If you lack sufficient flexibility, you can put a small block or a rolled carpet or towel under your heels.

Action
Maintain the position, allowing your pelvis to descend toward the floor, keeping your back relaxed.

Alternative
As you exhale, contract your transversus abdominis and pelvic floor muscles. As you inhale, expand your abdomen and back.

Visualization
Imagine that your coccyx (tailbone) is descending toward the floor.

AVOID	EFFECTS	DURATION
▸ Spreading your feet too far apart	▸ Increased suppleness in the lower back ▸ Greater mobility in the hips and knees ▸ Back pain relief	▸ 30 to 60 seconds

Lumbar spinal stretch (lying down)
▶ for all

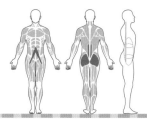

This exercise is a classic stretch for the lower back. In fact, people often do it instinctively. It is a simple exercise and can be done at any time. You can stretch your spinal muscles on both sides at the same time or one side at a time.

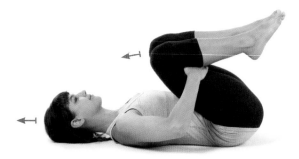

Bilateral Stretch

Initial Position

Lying on the back, knees bent, hands behind the thighs.

Action

Bring your thighs toward your abdomen. Maintain this position while breathing slowly and deeply.

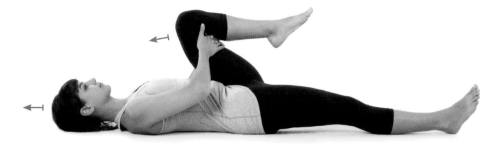

Unilateral Stretch

Action

Bring your thigh toward your abdomen. Maintain this position while breathing slowly and deeply. Repeat the exercise on the opposite side.

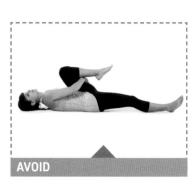

AVOID	EFFECTS	DURATION
▶ Extending your neck (use a cushion if needed to avoid)	▶ Increased suppleness in the lower back and hip flexors ▶ More efficient breathing ▶ Back pain relief	▶ 45 seconds

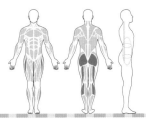

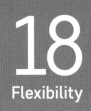

This exercise may cause some discomfort but is very effective for targeted areas. It stretches the gluteal, hamstring and fibularis muscles (lateral part of the leg). It also helps develop an ability to control movement between your pelvis and chest.

If you feel numbness, reduce the range of the stretch or stop the exercise immediately. You should not tolerate pain in the lower back, either.

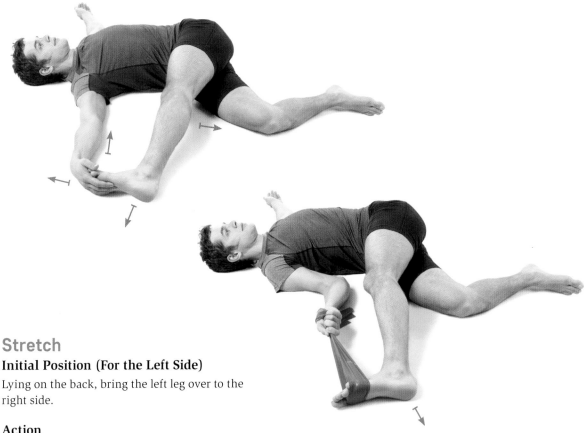

Stretch

Initial Position (For the Left Side)
Lying on the back, bring the left leg over to the right side.

Action
Extend your leg and bring it up toward your head as much as possible, then bring your toes (especially the big toe) toward you while pushing your heel away.

Repeat the exercise on the opposite side.

Beginner's Version
If you need help to hold your foot, use an elastic band or a towel, and keep the other knee bent.

AVOID	EFFECTS	DURATION
▸ Trying to flatten your back on the floor	▸ Increased suppleness in the posterolateral chain of the legs ▸ Greater mobility in the pelvis	▸ 45 seconds on each side

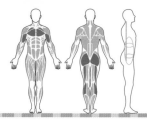

Some people have tense pectorals that draw their shoulders forward and round their back (kyphosis). Here is how to stretch the major and minor pectoral muscles. Some people try to build up their major pectoral muscles for aesthetic reasons, but these muscles (tonic muscles) tend to be tense naturally. The minor pectorals are the muscles that bring the shoulders forward. Too much tension in these muscles can also cause numbness in the forearms and hands. This exercise is strongly recommended for people who spend a lot of time in front of a computer.

In case of numbness in the fingers, reduce the range of the stretch. If numbness persists, hold the position for just 15 seconds. If the numbness is constant, consult a health-care professional.

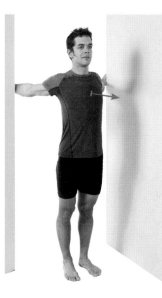

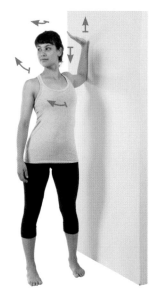

Major Pectoral

Initial Position
Standing, the hands behind a door frame.

Action
Move your trunk forward and breathe while trying to open up your sternum.

Minor Pectoral

Initial Position (For the Left Side)
Standing next to a wall, the feet in a comfortable position. The left arm is flattened against the wall, the elbow is level with the shoulder and the fingers are pulled down toward the floor.

Action
Once you are positioned, turn your head and trunk to the right, then roll your right shoulder backward and slightly upward to open your chest. Repeat the exercise on the opposite side.

AVOID
▶ Raising your arm too high
▶ Projecting your head forward

EFFECTS
▶ Increased suppleness in the pectorals
▶ Improved shoulder position
▶ More efficient breathing
▶ Better posture

DURATION
▶ 30 seconds (for each exercise)

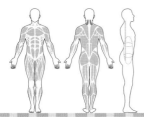
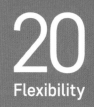
Just like the spinal muscles in the lower back, the cervical spinal muscles (in the neck) often need to be stretched. Here is how to do it in a bilateral fashion (both sides at once) and in a lateral fashion (one side at a time). As you would for the lower back, the ideal is to do a trio of stretches (start by unilateral stretching on both sides, then finish with the bilateral stretch). If you are short on time, just do the bilateral version.

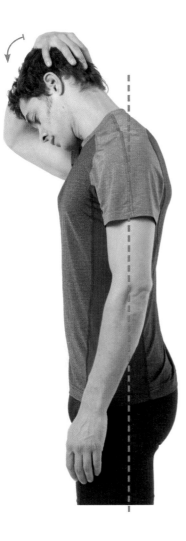

Bilateral Stretch

Initial Position

Standing or sitting, the back straight and the spinal column elongated, with one hand on top of the skull.

Action

Tilt your head forward toward your neck while slightly tucking in your chin, then tilt your neck forward toward the floor using your hand for assistance. Keep your back straight up to the junction between your shoulders and your neck. Maintain the position.

Unilateral Stretch

Action (For the Left Side)

Do the same thing but add a slight rotation of the neck to the right before tilting your head toward the floor.

Repeat the exercise on the opposite side.

AVOID	EFFECTS	DURATION
▸ Rounding the back	▸ Increased suppleness in the neck ▸ Neck pain relief	▸ 30 to 45 seconds in each position

Levator scapulae and upper trapezius stretch
▶ for all

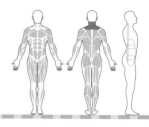

The levator scapulae is the muscle that raises the shoulder toward the head. It is often tense, especially in people who work at a computer terminal (such as our *homo sittingus*). Stretching the levator scapulae helps to ease neck pain and tension that radiates down into the shoulders. This exercise also stretches the upper trapezius, which tends to also be tense in most individuals.

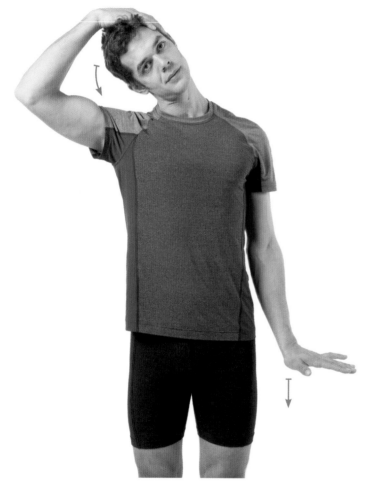

Initial Position (For the Left Side)
Sitting or standing, the right hand on the head, fingers on the left temple. The spinal column is stretched, the left arm is down, palm toward the floor and fingers pulled back.

Action
Push the heel of your left hand toward the floor, then tilt your head to the right and forward at the same time. Repeat the exercise on the opposite side.

AVOID	EFFECTS	DURATION
▶ Rounding your back ▶ Relaxing your palm that is pushing down toward the floor	▶ Increased suppleness in the neck ▶ Release of tension in the scapulae ▶ Relief of neck and head pain	▶ 45 seconds on each side

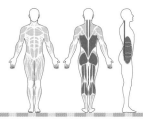

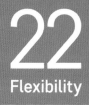

Highly recommended for easing pressure in the lower back, this exercise is ideal after a long day of walking or a long period spent standing or sitting. It encourages good blood flow from the lower limbs to the heart. This exercise should be done slowly, especially the first few times, as the lower back is not accustomed to relaxing in this position.

In case of numbness in the legs, reduce the tension in the elongation and hold the position for a shorter period of time (not more than 30 seconds). If the exercise continues to cause pain in your lower back, stop and consult a health-care professional.

Normal Version

Initial Position
Lying on the back, legs pressed against the wall. Place yourself as close to the wall as possible while keeping your pelvis pressed to the floor.

Action
1. Elongate the back of your neck and your spinal column.
2. Bring your toes toward the floor while pushing your heels toward the ceiling and your knees toward the wall.
3. With your arms stretched out on either side of your head, flex your wrists back and bring your fingers toward the wall. Maintain the position, breathing deeply.
4. Bend your knees and turn on your side to get up.

Pumping Version
You can also do abdominal pumps, which work deeply in the abdomen and lower back. As you inhale, expand your abdomen. As you exhale, pull your navel toward your spinal column.

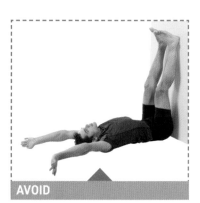

AVOID
▶ Placing your pelvis so close to the wall that your torso is no longer elongated and your legs tilt backward.
▶ Extending your neck

EFFECTS
▶ Reduced pressure in the lower back
▶ Back pain relief
▶ Greater flexibility in the posterior chain

DURATION
▶ 1 minute (you can also keep your legs raised for 1 to 2 minutes before doing the elongation. If you wish, add 5 abdominal pumps

Mobility

A gradual decline in back mobility is one of the consequences of daily life for many people. Mobility exercises need to be part of any back training program. By increasing the joints' capacity to move, these exercises also increase mobility in the spinal column (bending, stretching, rotating, leaning sideways and twisting), the chest (ribs and sternum), the hips and the thighs, all of which help the back to function properly. These exercises are also a good way to prepare your back for work that requires exertion.

The Key To Succeed

Once again, it does no good to strain your muscles. The most important thing is to respect your back and help it improve gradually. Remind yourself that your back has probably not moved this much in a very long time, so you need to give it time to adjust. You should try to move smoothly and without a lot of effort.

Duration

The recommended duration for these types of exercise is 30 to 60 seconds. You can also count the number of repetitions, which is ideally between 10 and 20.

Caution

If you already feel pain, do the movements slowly and reduce the range so you do not increase the pain. Take extra care to relax and breathe deeply. Mobility exercises should never increase pain, either during or after.

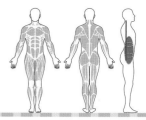

Here is a basic exercise familiar to anyone who practices yoga or Pilates. It helps to improve the back's ability to bend and stretch and is safe if performed correctly. The basic idea is not to strain as well as to use your breathing to mobilize your back.

Alternate from one position to the next in a smooth fashion, without a lot of effort, keeping your neck extended in a line from your back.

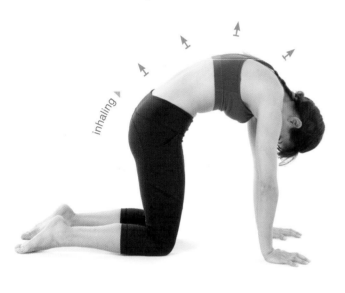

inhaling

Cat Pose

Initial Position

Starting on all fours, with the head extended in a straight line from the back, which remains neutral, hands under the shoulders and knees under the hips.

Action

Tilt your pelvis by directing your pubic bone toward your navel (visualize a tail hanging downward).

Hold your head extended straight from your back.

As you inhale, round your back while trying to expand it.

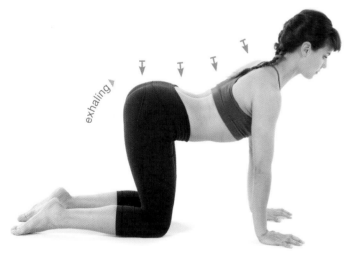

exhaling

Cow Pose

Action

Tilt your pelvis by directing your pubic bone downward (visualize a tail rising upward).

Hold your head extended straight from your back.

As you exhale, hollow your back without making an effort by exhaling and not by forcing your back muscles.

AVOID	EFFECTS	DURATION
▶ Stretching your neck ▶ Bending your elbows	▶ Greater mobility and elasticity in the back ▶ More efficient breathing ▶ Back pain relief	▶ 10 to 20 repetitions

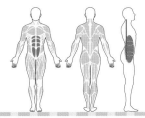

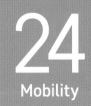

You can hold each position for 30 seconds and practice holding your breath, which also helps to develop flexibility and breathing.

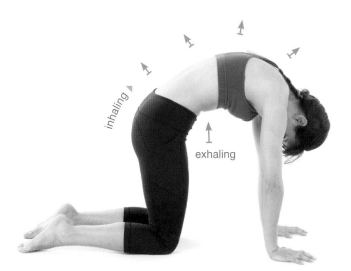

inhaling

exhaling

Cat Pose

Initial Position

Same position as in the previous exercise.

Action

As you inhale, expand your back. As you exhale, pull in your navel toward your spinal column as if you were pushing from the inside to round your back.

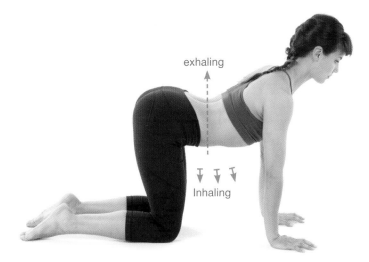

exhaling

Inhaling

Cow Pose

Action

As you inhale, expand your abdomen. As you exhale, pull in your navel toward your spinal column, keeping your back hollow.

AVOID	EFFECTS	DURATION
▸ Straining to maintain the position	▸ Greater mobility and elasticity in the back ▸ More efficient breathing ▸ Back pain relief	▸ 1 to 3 cycles (1 cycle = 5 breaths in one position + 5 in the other position)

25

Mobility

Tail wag
▶ for all

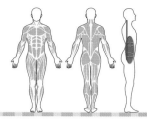

This exercise relaxes the back by targeting lateral (sideways) bending. It is part of a more complete routine done in the all-fours position. The key to succeed is to move energetically but effortlessly. The alternative Cat/Cow poses are also easy and effective. This is a popular exercise that I frequently recommend.

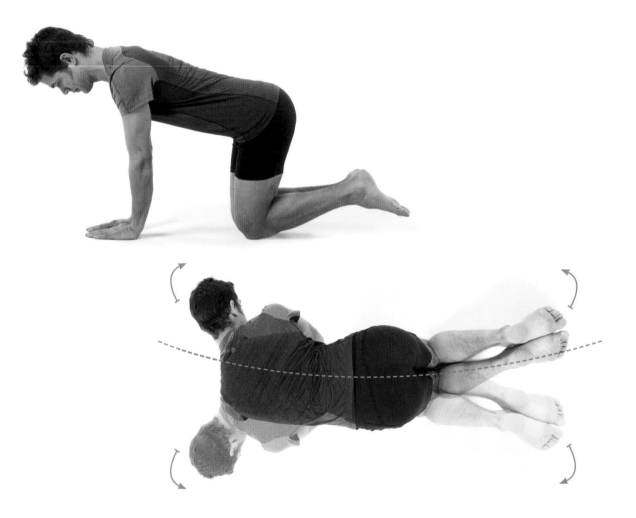

Normal Version

Initial Position

Starting on all fours, with hands and knees parallel and feet slightly raised.

Action

In a rhythmic fashion, tilt your feet and head at the same time to one side, alternating from side to side.

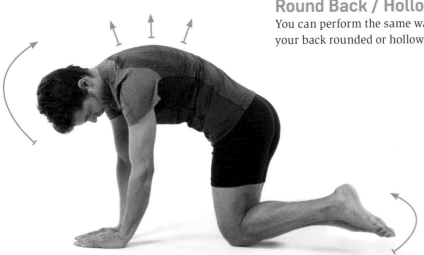

Round Back / Hollow Back Alternatives

You can perform the same wagging movement, keeping your back rounded or hollow, without straining.

Tip

You can alternate from one position to another without stopping the wagging movement (example: back neutral for 15 seconds + rounded back for 15 seconds + hollow back for 15 seconds + neutral back for 15 seconds).

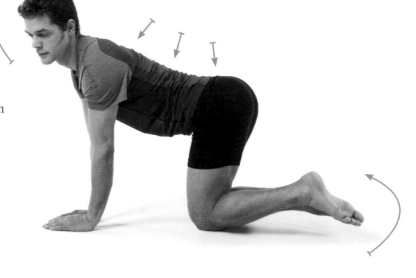

AVOID	EFFECTS	DURATION
▸ Jerky or forced movements	▸ Greater mobility in the back ▸ Back pain relief	▸ 30 to 60 seconds

Cat stretch
▶ for all

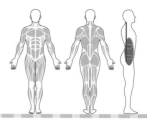

The Cat Stretch is a more dynamic version of the Cat/Cow pose. It helps increase mobility in the back, pelvis and hips. As it requires a certain amount of coordination, take the time to master this feline movement. The key word here is "fluidity."

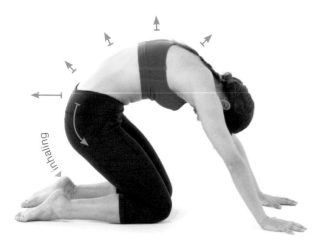

inhaling

Rounded Back to the Back
Initial Position
Starting on all fours.

Action
As you inhale, gradually round your back and move your body toward your feet.

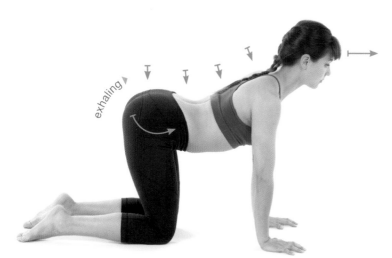

exhaling

Hollow Back To the Front
Action
As you exhale, gradually hollow your back and move your body toward your hands.

These two positions should work together as one fluid, continuous movement, like the turning of a wheel.

The Key To Succeed
Find a way to tilt your pelvis that will allow you to make a smooth transition between the rounded back and hollow back positions.

AVOID
▶ Stiffening your pelvis
▶ Bending your elbows (keep your elbows extended to help target the back)

EFFECTS
▶ Greater mobility in the back, pelvis and hips
▶ More efficient breathing
▶ Back pain relief

DURATION
▶ 10 repetitions, keeping the movement fluid

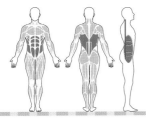
The Back Twist is a key exercise for the back and one I often recommend to my patients. It allows the spinal column to turn more easily and helps to mobilize the chest, including the ribs and sternum.

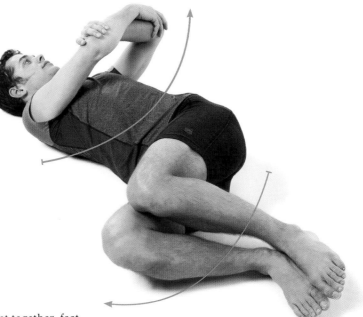

Initial Position

Lying on the back, the knees bent and kept together, feet together, hands on the opposite elbows.

Action

As you inhale, turn your head and arms to one side while turning your knees to the opposite side. As you exhale, bring your arms and knees to the center, using your core muscles (transversus abdominis and pelvic floor). Repeat the exercise on the opposite side.

The Key To Succeed

The movement should be fluid and without added strain.

AVOID	EFFECTS	DURATION
▸ Twisting too far in the opposite direction	▸ Greater mobility in the spinal column, chest and pelvis ▸ More efficient breathing ▸ Back pain relief	▸ 10 repetitions on each side

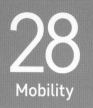

28
Mobility

Back twist (advanced)
▸ intermediate to advanced

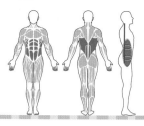

Derived from an osteopathic technique, this more elaborate version of the back twist develops the ability to dissociate movement between the pelvis, chest, skull, eyes and even the tongue. The last movement is fun but it also has a purpose.

Turning the head in the opposite direction toward the arms helps target the base of the neck and upper chest. This is an excellent exercise for people who have tension in these areas. Adding eye movement to the exercise helps work the base of the skull. Finally, adding the tongue to the exercise helps activate the muscular chain that includes the tongue, esophagus and stomach. For many individuals, this last step helps disengage the back muscles due to the muscular chain's numerous connections to the spinal column. The tongue is connected to the base of the skull and the neck, and the esophagus is connected to the upper chest.

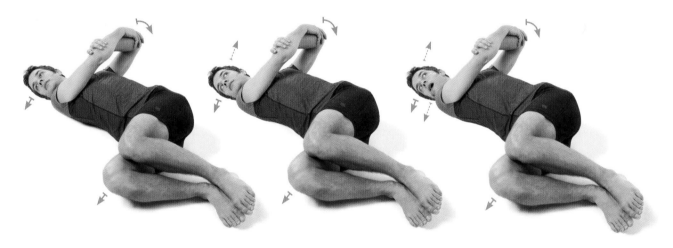

Pelvis-Chest-Neck Twist
Initial Position
Same position as in Exercise 27.

Action
Like the standard twist, but turning the head in the opposite direction of the arms.

Pelvis-Chest-Neck-Eyes Twist
Action
Like the previous twist, but turning the eyes in the opposite direction of the head.

Pelvis-Chest-Neck-Eyes-Tongue Twist
Action
Like the previous twist, but pushing the tongue in the opposite direction of the eyes.

AVOID
▸ Twisting too far in the opposite direction

EFFECTS
▸ Greater mobility in the spinal column, chest and pelvis
▸ More efficient breathing
▸ Back pain relief

DURATION
▸ 5 repetitions on each side, for each version

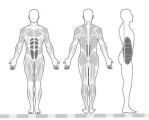

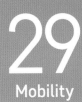
Too many people have a rigid pelvis. This exercise helps to mobilize the pelvis and is a basic component in many other movements and exercises.

Forward Pelvic Tilt

Initial Position

Lying on the back, knees bent, feet and knees aligned with the hips and the back neutral.

Action

As you exhale, bring your pubic bone toward your feet and let your lower back slowly arch.

As you inhale, return to the neutral position.

Note: The photo shows the hands raised for a better view of the pelvis but it is not required to raise them.

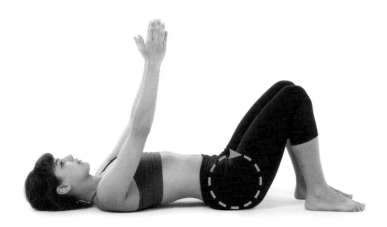

Backward Pelvic Tilt

Action

As you exhale, bring your pubic bone toward your navel and your navel toward your spinal column while flattening your lower back against the floor. As you inhale, return to the neutral position.

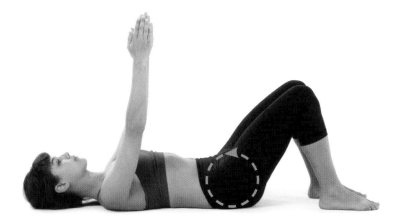

AVOID

▸ Flattening your lower back without tilting your pelvis when doing the backward pelvic tilt
▸ Straining to arch your back

EFFECTS

▸ Greater mobility and more control of the pelvis

DURATION

▸ 10 repetitions

Prune face/Baby lion face
▶ for all

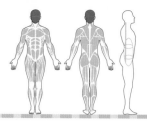

Do not judge the effectiveness of the exercise by its name. The Prune Face/Baby Lion Face is an excellent exercise for relaxing the muscles of the face and head. Recommended for tension in the jaw, eyes and neck (especially at the base of the skull), this entertaining exercise also has a relaxing effect on the nervous system. Do it in private and on your own or as a couple if you have a rock-solid ego.

This exercise is especially recommended for people who work at a computer terminal or for people who accumulate a lot of tension in the face and jaw.

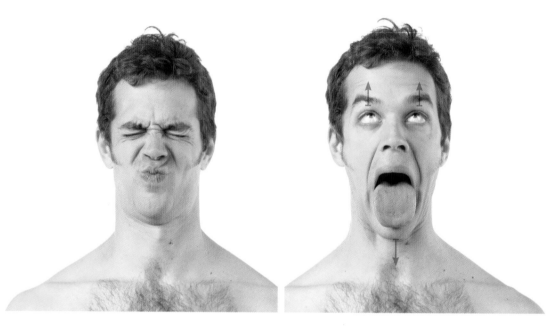

Prune Face

Initial Position

Sitting or standing.

Action

As you exhale, contract all your facial muscles by scrunching your forehead, eyes, cheeks, nose, mouth and chin.

Baby Lion Face

Action

As you inhale, open your mouth wide, stick out your tongue and extend it downward as far as possible while turning your eyes upward. Keep your head level.

AVOID

▶ Excess straining

EFFECTS

▶ Relaxation of the muscles in the face, head and neck

DURATION

▶ 5 repetitions, alternating the Prune Face and Baby Lion Face

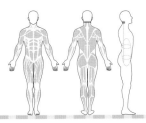
Here is the best exercise for relaxing the suboccipital muscles at the base of the skull. It's tricky to "break" the oculomotor reflex (see "The Neck-Eyes Link" on page 55) by turning your eyes in the opposite direction of your neck. This exercise is recommended if you work a lot at your computer. It can be done standing or sitting, while maintaining good posture. Do the neck rotation exercises first, followed by the neck flexion and extension exercise.

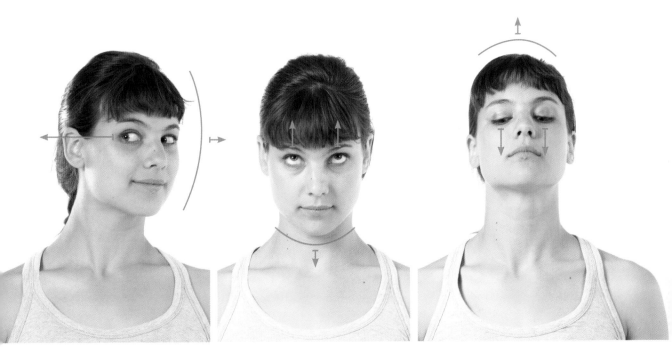

Neck Rotation ("No" Movement)

Initial Position

Sitting or standing, facing forward.

Action

As you exhale, turn your head 45 degrees to one side, slowly and gently, while looking in the opposite direction.

As you inhale, bring your head and your eyes back to the center. Repeat the exercise on the opposite side.

Neck Flexion and Extension ("Yes" Movement)

Action

As you exhale, lower your head slightly while looking upward. As you inhale, raise your head slowly back to its normal position and look forward.

As you exhale, raise your head (and chin) slightly while looking downward. As you inhale, lower your head slowly back to its normal position and look forward.

AVOID	EFFECTS	DURATION
▸ Turning your head more than 45 degrees	▸ Relaxation of the muscles at the base of the skull, neck and head	▸ 5 neck rotations on each side, followed by 5 flexion and extension movements

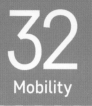

32
Mobility

Neck figure 8's
▶ for all

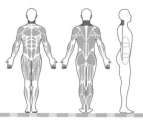

This is by far the best and safest exercise for relaxing the neck. What's more, it doesn't require much effort. All you need is to make 8 horizontal figure 8's (∞ like the infinity sign) and 8 vertical figure 8's with some simple head movements that activate all of the neck muscles at the same time. A smaller horizontal 8 targets more of the neck muscles while more muscles are engaged with a vertical 8. Personally, it is my favorite exercise to do in front of the computer. I have fun by switching from a vertical 8 to a horizontal 8 at random in a fluid routine. It instantly relaxes the neck.

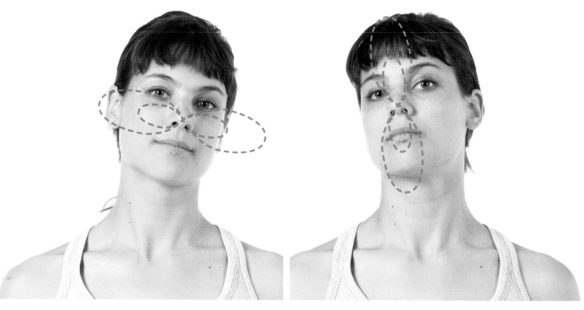

Horizontal ∞

Initial Position
Sitting or standing, facing forward.

Action
Imagine that you have paint on your nose and that you want to use it to trace a small horizontal ∞ on a sheet of paper in front of you. In a slow, fluid motion, tilt your head to make the small figure 8.

Vertical 8

Action
The same as for the previous exercise, but tracing a vertical figure 8.

The Key To Succeed
Aim for slow, effortless and fluid movement while gazing forward.

To target your upper neck, make small figure 8's.

A larger figure 8 activates a larger portion of the spinal column.

AVOID	EFFECTS	DURATION
▶ Straining to do the movements or making the range of movement too large ▶ Gazing at your nose while "painting"	▶ Relaxation of the neck muscles ▶ Neck pain relief ▶ Greater mobility in the neck	▶ 5 to 10 repetitions in each direction for the horizontal ∞ and the vertical 8

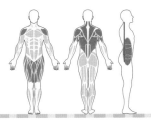

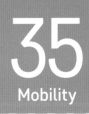
This is a very good exercise to fight the tendency to slump when we are sitting. Much of the tension in the back is relieved while it regains its ability to lengthen.

Do this exercise gradually. Some people have difficulty doing a full movement toward the ceiling. This may be due to insufficient mobility in the back and perhaps the shoulders. In this case, reduce the range of movement. This exercise is recommended for people who spend a lot of time sitting.

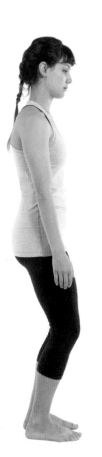

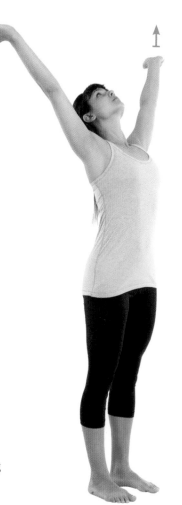

Initial Position
Standing, knees slightly bent and the back relaxed.

Action
As you inhale, raise your arms up, push the palms of your hands upward, tilt your head slighly back and look toward the ceiling. As you exhale, return to the initial position.

Visualization
Imagine your spinal column remaining lengthened throughout the movement.

AVOID	EFFECTS	DURATION
▸ Extending your neck too much	▸ Greater mobility in the back and shoulders ▸ Better posture ▸ Back pain relief	▸ 5 to 10 repetitions

Breathing

When was the last time you breathed freely and in a relaxed manner? The exercises presented here will help you get back in touch with your breathing, and in a way, with yourself. If you have difficulty with these exercises, try them in the evening after an exhausting physical activity. Give yourself time to master this aspect of movement. You'll be surprised at the results over the long term.

The Key To Succeed

Natural, effortless breathing.

Duration

Each exercise can be done for about 1 minute, but you can also do them for longer (up to 20 minutes) and benefit from the relaxation they provide. Be aware of your body's sensations and take the time to breathe properly.

Caution

Some people are uncomfortable doing meditation, relaxation or breathing exercises, preferring instead those activities in which a lot of energy is expended, such as running or tennis. Breathing exercises may seem like they are not for everyone — they require going inside yourself and being aware of your bodily sensations. Breathing says a lot about your internal state and this can be distressing for some people. If this is the case, I can suggest two ways to make it easier. The first is to do the abdominal breathing exercises while doing your favorite activity. Breathing this way while running is especially good. The second way, which is more difficult, is to work on your weak spot and try to do one breathing exercise every day for one week.

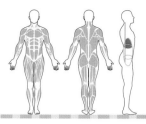

This exercise does wonders for releasing stress when it is bottled up. It is highly recommended for people who hyperventilate a lot or have difficulty exhaling. People who have asthma, for example, can also benefit from this breathing exercise. The principle is simple but the exercise is not easy. You have to breathe slowly and a little more deeply than you would normally. At the end of the exhalation, wait for the inhalation to come all by itself in an involuntary fashion.

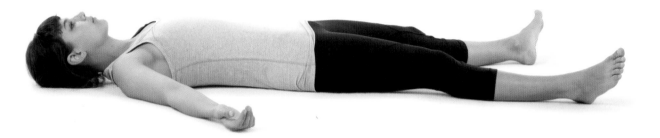

Initial Position

Lying on the back, allow the entire body to sink into the floor.

Action

1. Exhaling: Blow the air through your mouth, with your lips relaxed, emptying your lungs slowly, and a little more than usual. Do not strain.

2. Relaxation: This is the "release" part of the exercise. Instead of intentionally inhaling right away, wait for the inhalation to come by itself, naturally, without any intention or effort.

3. Inhaling: Inhale through your nose, as naturally as possible, without trying to control anything. Trust your body.

AVOID	EFFECTS	DURATION
▸ Straining to exhale	▸ More efficient breathing ▸ Lowered response to stress ▸ Back pain relief	▸ 1 to 3 minutes or 5 to 15 breaths

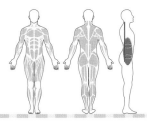
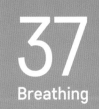
This exercise, which is excellent for mobilizing the thoracic diaphragm, helps you learn proper abdominal and sternal breathing. Both are necessary but some people have more difficulty with one over the other.

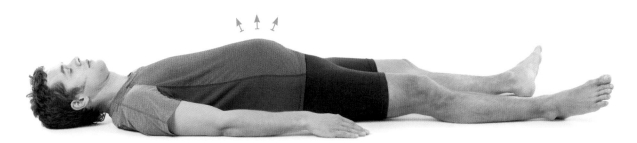

Abdominal Breathing

Initial Position
Lying on the back.

Action
As you inhale, let your abdomen expand slowly, without effort. As you exhale, relax your abdomen.

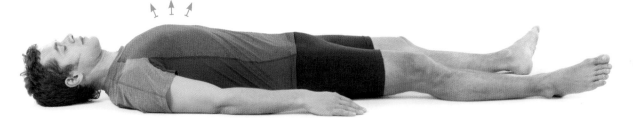

Sternal Breathing

Action
As you inhale, let your sternum rise slowly, without effort.

As you exhale, imagine that your sternum is becoming soft and sinking to the floor and down to your feet.

Tip
Once you have mastered both ways of breathing, you can combine the two for fuller and more natural breathing. It is normal for the sternum to have more difficulty moving than the abdomen. The abdomen is more elastic, while movement in the sternum is limited by the mobility of the chest, which is made up of many different bones.

The Key To Succeed
Your back should remain relaxed. Do not arch it or try flattening it into the floor.

AVOID	EFFECTS	DURATION
▸ Arching your back to expand your abdomen	▸ More efficient breathing ▸ Back pain relief	▸ 5 to 10 breaths of each type

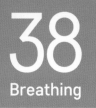

Deep exhalation
▶ for all

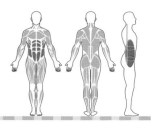

This is an ideal exercise for people who are chronically stressed. It requires that you exhale explosively, that is, deeply and quickly at the same time, working the abdominal muscles. This technique has some great benefits. First, it relaxes the diaphragm. Second, it expells a lot of the residual air in the lungs (that is, from the stagnant part of the lung that does not work as hard). Third, it helps encourage blood flow to all parts of the body. This exercise is useful for relaxing your back, which may experience stiffness because of a very tense diaphragm. It is not advisable, however, for people suffering from a herniated disk or if you are in pain due to sneezing or coughing.

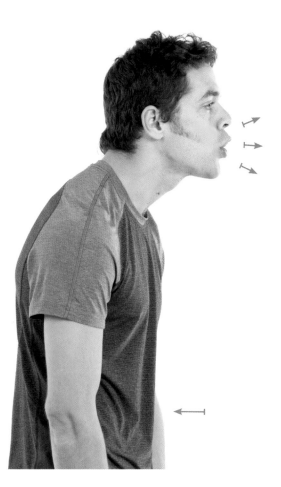

Initial Position
Standing or sitting.

Action
Exhale in an explosive fashion, then inhale slowly and deeply. Your muscles should contract naturally while you exhale.

AVOID	EFFECTS	DURATION
▶ Closing your mouth often, which doesn't allow the air you're breathing out to escape easily	▶ Relaxation of the thoracic diaphragm ▶ Release of back tension ▶ Encouraging blood flow	▶ 3 to 5 repetitions

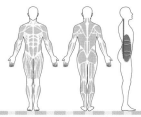

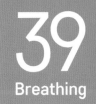

This three-step breathing exercise helps to rebalance the nervous system.

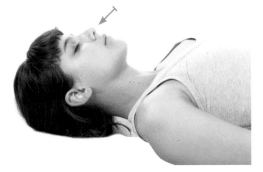

Inhaling

Initial Position
Lying on the back.

Action
Inhale through your nose and hold your breath for 10 seconds.

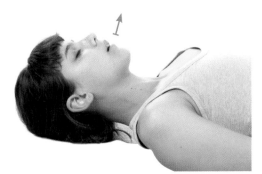

Exhaling

Action
Exhale through your mouth and hold your breath for 10 seconds.

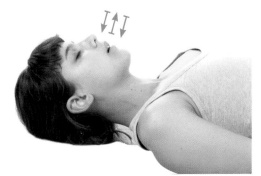

Panting

Action
Alternate inhaling and exhaling by panting (like a dog) for 10 seconds.

Tip
You can settle for one cycle (inhaling + exhaling + panting) for a duration of 30 seconds. For best results, breathe normally for 10 seconds between each cycle and do 3 cycles.

AVOID	EFFECTS	DURATION
▸ Inhaling or exhaling too deeply	▸ More efficient breathing ▸ Rebalanced nervous system ▸ Back pain relief	▸ 1 to 3 times for each cycle

Child's pose
▶ for all

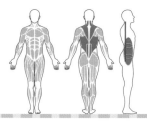

This pose, which has been adopted by yoga, Pilates and other fitness regimens, has a relaxing effect on the whole body. It is an essential exercise that gives your body a break, lets you reconnect with the earth and helps you breathe using your back. It should be avoided if you have a herniated disk.

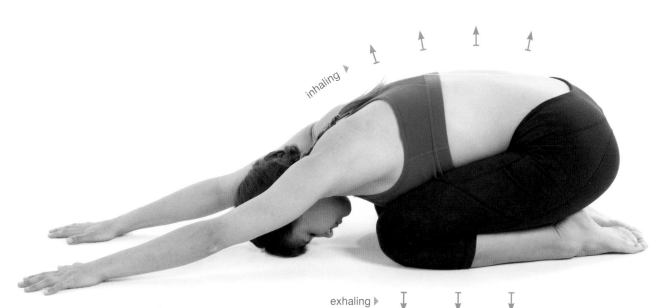

inhaling ▶

exhaling ▶

Initial Position

Kneeling, letting the entire body sink to the floor while your arms stretch out in front of your head.

Action

As you inhale, slowly expand your back. As you exhale, flatten your back and relax your arms above your shoulders as you imagine your entire body sinking into the ground.

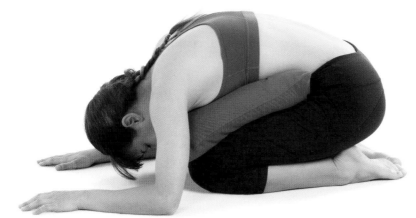

Version with a Cushion

To help open up the back, place a cushion on your knees and repeat Exercise 40 but rest your chest on the pillow and bend your elbows while bringing your body to the floor.

Version with a Support Under the Head

For people who cannot rest their head on the floor, place a cushioned support under your head while repeating Exercise 40. Bring your hands to the side to hold the support in place.

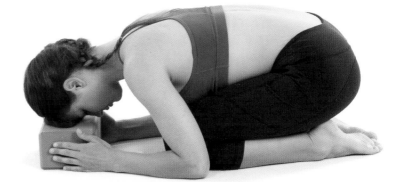

AVOID	EFFECTS	DURATION
▸ Straining to press against the floor	▸ More efficient breathing ▸ Back pain relief ▸ Rebalanced nervous system	▸ 1 to 2 minutes or 5 to 10 breaths

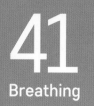

41

Breathing

Pumping abdominal twist

▶ for all

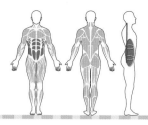

This exercise is recommended for the diaphragm and the back. It has a positive effect on all of the organs in the abdomen and chest. People who suffer from inflammatory digestive diseases (for eg., Crohn's disease) should do this exercise slowly. In the right dose, it can provide some relief. This exercise is effective for back problems associated with difficulty digesting or eliminating and for reproductive system problems.

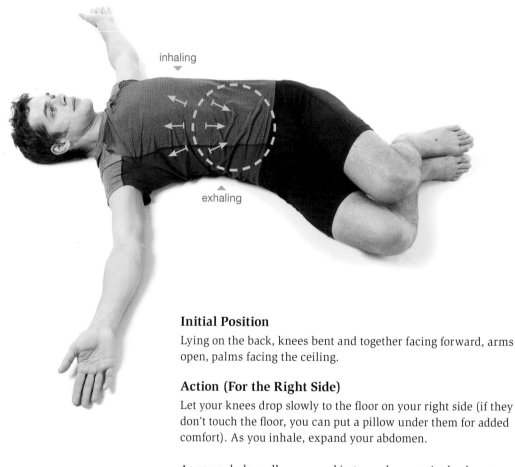

inhaling

exhaling

Initial Position

Lying on the back, knees bent and together facing forward, arms open, palms facing the ceiling.

Action (For the Right Side)

Let your knees drop slowly to the floor on your right side (if they don't touch the floor, you can put a pillow under them for added comfort). As you inhale, expand your abdomen.

As you exhale, pull your navel in toward your spinal column. Repeat the exercise on your left side.

AVOID	EFFECTS	DURATION
▶ Straining to bring your legs too far	▶ Greater mobility in the lower back and abdomen ▶ More efficient breathing ▶ Improved digestion ▶ Back pain relief	▶ 5 breaths on each side

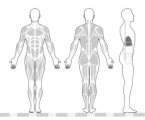
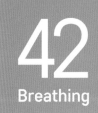
Marvelous for some, torture for others, this exercise leaves no one indifferent. It is designed to relax your thoracic diaphragm through pressure from your fingers. This fairly unpleasant technique also relaxes the zone of the liver, the stomach and the solar plexus (which are often very tense). Place your fingers under your ribs as though you were palpating the insides of your ribs. Be careful not to push your fingers in too deeply, as you will be pressing directly on your organs, which is not good.

You have to do this exercise slowly at first in order to get comfortable with it. If it causes discomfort, stop.

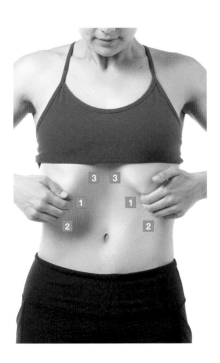

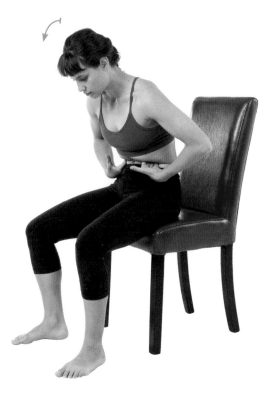

Initial Position

Sitting, the fingers (except for the thumbs) just under the ribs, in Position 1.

Action

Lean forward and place your fingers under your ribs. Inhale and maintain the pressure of your fingers (this prevents your diaphragm from dropping). Exhale and let your fingers move inward if your tissues allow them. Do not force them. Begin again, leaving your fingers in Position 2, and then in Position 3.

AVOID

▸ Pushing your fingers into your abdomen. You should reach under your ribs to touch your diaphragm

EFFECTS

▸ Relaxation of the thoracic diaphragm
▸ More efficient breathing
▸ Back pain relief

DURATION

▸ 3 repetitions in each position

Posture

Postural exercises are of the utmost importance for the health of your back. Since we have already devoted a whole chapter to posture, we will now focus entirely on some original exercises that I call helical elongations, or helicals. Being quite novel and also subtle, helical elongations require a great deal of concentration, especially at the beginning. Give yourself time to master these new movements, which will do you a world of good.

The Keys To Succeed

When doing helical elongation exercises, think of the body (the pelvis in particular) as a bottle and the spinal column as the cork. Here are the steps to optimizing results when doing the following exercises:

- Hold the bottle (the pelvis) down firmly in order to pull out the cork (the spinal column). This downward force helps the helical to move upward. Keep the knees slightly bent. The pelvis should neither rise nor turn during an helical.
- Pull the cork (the spinal column) upward while turning. You are trying to grow taller (elongation) while slightly turning your head and trunk.
- Pull the top of your skull toward the ceiling while looking toward the horizon (do not look up or down).
- Pull out the cork during inhalation. During exhaling, allow the cork to return to normal. Do helicals on both sides, first to the right, then to the left, alternating between the two.

Repetitions

Five to 10 repetitions are sufficient for the helical elongation exercise. If you can do several, five repetitions on each side will largely suffice. For the other postural exercises, see the recommendations in the exercise description.

Caution

Once again, these exercises should not be accompanied by pain, during or after, but this is rarely the case for this type of exercise. Postural exercises require a good deal of concentration. Therefore, it is not recommended that you do them while watching television, for example.

Bounces
▶ for all

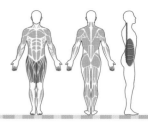

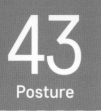

This exercise restores energy and is an excellent way to prepare your body for physical activity. Use it as a warm-up before a workout or to wake up after an afternoon break. It is designed to stimulate the deep muscles of the spinal column and to activate the quadriceps, which will help you maintain good posture. The principle is simple: Bounce in a loose and rhythmic way.

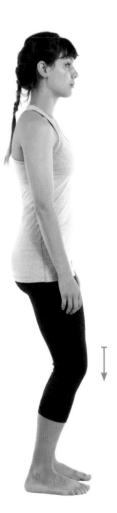

Knee Flexion

Initial Position

Standing, jaw relaxed, shoulders relaxed, back straight and spinal column elongated.

Action

Lower your body slightly.

Knee Extension

Action

Stand up quickly.

The Key To Succeed

Maintain your energy while remaining relaxed. Bounce in an energetic way. At the end of the exercise, your thighs should feel warm.

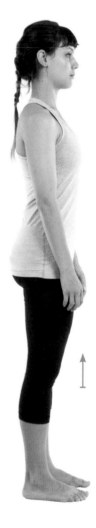

AVOID

▶ Moving too slowly and mechanically

EFFECTS

▶ Activation of the postural muscles
▶ Muscle warm-up
▶ Energized nervous system

DURATION

▶ 30 seconds

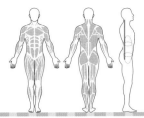

The deep spinal muscles in the dorsal region often weaken and fail to do their job in helping you maintain proper posture. This exercise is a good way to stimulate these muscles, particularly the small muscles connected from one vertebra to the next. This exercise can be done at the computer from time to time. Ten seconds is enough to make a difference.

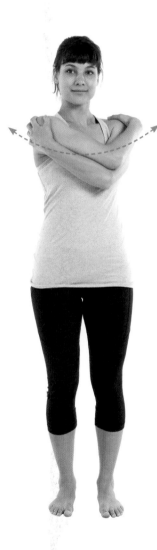

Initial Position

Sitting on the buttock or standing, firmly grounded, spinal column elongated, arms crossed to touch the scapulae (shoulder blades).

Action

Turn slightly (about 15 degrees) from one side to the other, in an energetic way, without forcing it, keeping your spinal column elongated, for 15 seconds, then switch the position of your arms and repeat.

AVOID	EFFECTS	DURATION
▸ Doing the movement too slowly	▸ Activation of the deep muscles of the spinal column ▸ Better posture ▸ Back pain relief	▸ 15 seconds in each position

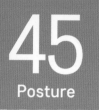

Balancing on one leg
▶ for all

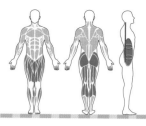

Balancing on one leg is a key element in many exercise programs. It helps improve your balance by activating the proprioceptors in a significant way. No matter what your level of activity, this exercise can help you. The key is to use the principles of grounding and elongation to improve its efficacy. To obtain better balance, strong legs and proper posture, this simple exercise is a must!

With elongation and grounding, the postural muscles are activated in the right way and balancing on one leg is easier.

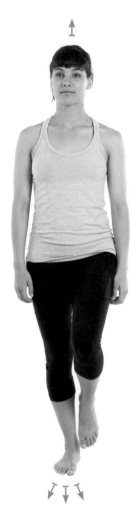

Initial Position
Standing.

Action
Stay balanced on one leg. This exercise can be done in several ways. You can start by leaning against the wall, and then without support, and then finally with your eyes closed (advanced level only).

Visualization
1. Imagine that a small string attached to the top of your skull is slowly pulling your head toward the ceiling. This string is keeping your entire body balanced.
2. Imagine roots growing from your toes, heels and the balls of your feet into the ground.

AVOID	EFFECTS	DURATION
▶ Slouching	▶ Better balance ▶ Increased proprioception ▶ Better posture ▶ Strengthening the lower limbs ▶ Greater stability	▶ 1 to 2 minutes on each foot

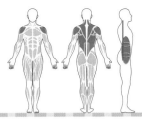

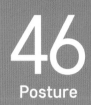

Inspired by a yoga pose, this exercise activates the mid-chest area (between the scapulae). It is recommended for people who spend a lot of time sitting. It should be done gradually. The first few times, you may feel the muscles working deeply between the scapulae, even for several hours after doing the exercise.

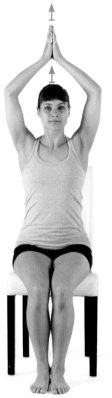

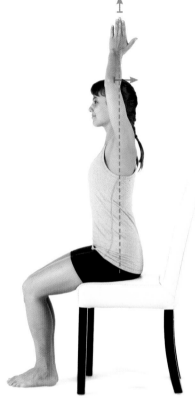

Initial Position

Sitting on the floor with weight balanced on the buttocks, back straight, spinal column aligned (people who are not able to keep their back straight sitting cross-legged can put a fairly large, stable block under the buttocks, or sit on a chair), hands above the head, palms together, fingers pointing toward the ceiling.

Action

Bring your elbows back so that your hips, shoulders, elbows, hands and ears are aligned when viewed from the side. Elongate the back of your neck. Extend the top of your head and stretch your hands toward the ceiling at the same time. Hold the position.

The Key To Succeed

Keep your spinal column elongated.

AVOID

▸ Letting your head drop forward
▸ Curving your back
▸ Bringing your elbows too far back
▸ Losing your alignment

EFFECTS

▸ Better posture
▸ Strengthening the deep muscles of the back

DURATION

▸ 30 to 60 seconds

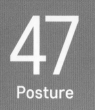

47

Posture

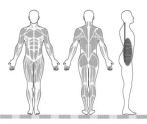

Helical elongation of the back
▸ for all

This first exercise in the helical series activates the entire spinal column and is a good preparation for the rest of the exercises in the series. If you are only going to do one exercise for posture, this is a good one to choose.

Initial Position
Standing, feet aligned with the hips, knees slightly bent.

Action
As you inhale, extend the top of your head toward the ceiling while turning slowly. Your trunk and spinal column rotate to follow the direction of your head. Your pelvis should not move.

As you exhale, return to the starting position, allowing your spinal column to resume to its normal length. Change direction.

The Key To Succeed
Imagine you are growing taller while slightly turning your head and trunk. The rotation should not be too pronounced.

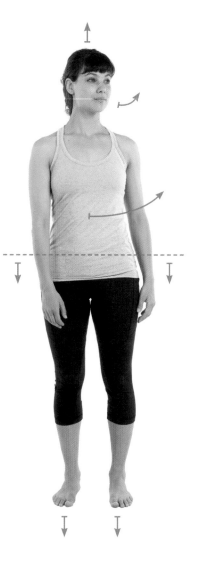

AVOID	EFFECTS	DURATION
▸ Losing the alignment of your head ▸ Straightening (extending) your knees ▸ Allowing your shoulders to rise	▸ Better posture ▸ Activation of the deep muscles of the spinal column and the core muscles	▸ 5 to 10 repetitions in each direction

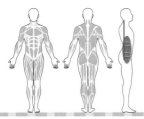
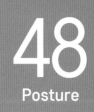
Stretching your arms downward in this way targets the cervical muscles of your neck. This exercise is recommended for people who have a sore or compressed neck.

If you feel numbness in the hands, reduce the tension in your palms. If the numbness continues, stop the exercise immediately.

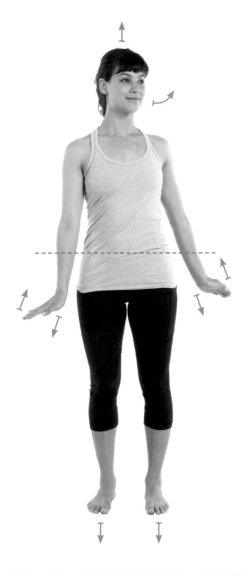

Initial Position

Standing, feet aligned with the hips, knees slightly bent, palms pushed downward and fingers pulled upward.

Action

As you inhale, extend the top of your head toward the ceiling while turning your head slowly. Your trunk and spinal column should rotate to follow the movement of your head. Your pelvis should not move.

As you exhale, return to the starting position, allowing your spinal column to resume to its normal length. Change direction.

The Key To Succeed

Keep your palms facing the floor during the entire exercise.

AVOID	EFFECTS	DURATION
▸ Losing the alignment of your head ▸ Straightening (extending) your knees ▸ Raising your shoulders	▸ Better posture ▸ Activation of the deep muscles of the spinal column and the core muscles ▸ Loosening of the neck muscles	▸ 5 to 10 repetitions in each direction

Helical elongation of the lumbar muscles
▸ for all

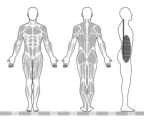

Raising your hands over your head targets your lower back, making this a good exercise for most people.

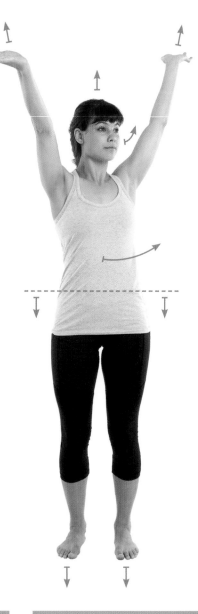

Initial Position

Standing, feet aligned with the hips, knees slightly bent, pushing the palms upward and pulling the fingers downward. The shoulders should remain low.

Action

As you inhale, extend the top of your head toward the ceiling while turning your head slowly. Your trunk and spinal column rotate to follow the movement of your head. Your pelvis should not move.

As you exhale, return to the starting position, allowing your spinal column to resume its normal length. Change direction.

AVOID

▸ Losing the alignment of your head
▸ Straightening (extending) your knees
▸ Raising your shoulders

EFFECTS

▸ Better posture
▸ Activation of the deep muscles of the spinal column and the core muscles
▸ Release of the lower back

DURATION

▸ 5 to 10 repetitions in each direction

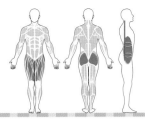

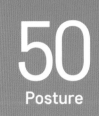
The helical elongation with a lunge is a full and challenging postural exercise. Maintaining the lunge is a challenge in itself, and working the deep muscles of the spinal column at the same time makes it a harder workout. The most difficult part is to hold the lunge position without lifting your pelvis. It is a marvelous way to awaken the deep muscles of the back and the legs.

Initial Position

In the Lunge position (see page 185), feet aligned with the hips, pelvis straight, facing forward and the knee over the foot. The thigh is held as horizontally as possible, the back is straight and the back leg extended.

Action

As you inhale, extend the top of your head toward the ceiling while slowly turning your head. Your trunk and spinal column rotate to follow the movement of your head. Your pelvis should not move.

As you exhale, return to the starting position, allowing your spinal column to resume its normal length. Repeat the action in the opposite direction.

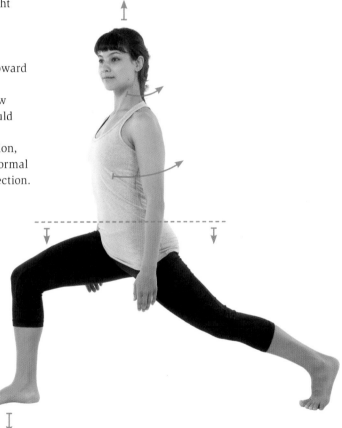

AVOID	EFFECTS	DURATION
▸ Losing the alignment of your head ▸ Abandoning the lunge position ▸ Raising your shoulders	▸ Better posture ▸ Activation and strengthening of the deep muscles of the spinal column, core muscles and lower limbs	▸ 5 to 10 repetitions on each side

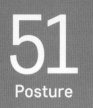

Helical elongation on one leg
▶ intermediate to advanced

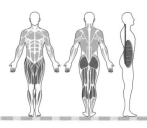

Here, we bring in one more element to the helical elongation — balancing on one leg. This exercise helps to work the muscles of the supporting lower limb (the limb you are standing on) in a spiral movement. You will be surprised to feel the deep muscles in your feet and your buttocks being activated.

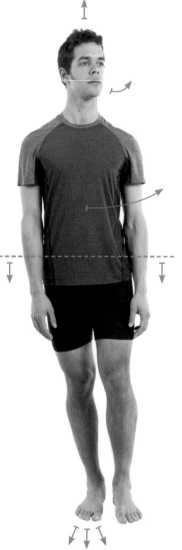

Initial Position
Balancing on one leg.

Action
As you inhale, extend the top of your head toward the ceiling while slowly turning your head. Your trunk and spinal column rotate to follow the movement of your head. You can let your pelvis turn as well.

As you exhale, return to the initial position, allowing your spinal column to resume its normal length. Change direction. Repeat the exercise on the other leg.

AVOID
▶ Losing the alignment of your head and back
▶ Raising your shoulders

EFFECTS
▶ Better posture
▶ Better balance
▶ Activation and strengthening of the deep muscles of the spinal column, the core muscles and the lower limbs

DURATION
▶ 5 to 10 repetitions in each direction, on each leg

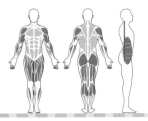
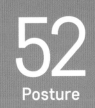
This exercise is more challenging than the other helical elongations. The others need to be mastered before you attempt this exercise, which adds spiral movements in the upper and lower limbs to activate the spinal column. This exercise requires a high degree of control.

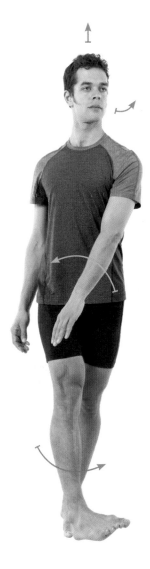

Initial Position
Balancing on one leg.

Action
As you inhale, raise your left arm to the height of your eyes, turning your thumb outward, while raising your right leg and bringing your little toe backward. Your head pivots to the left following the elongation in your left arm.

As you exhale, bring your left arm down, turning your thumb inward, while lowering your right leg and turning your large toe inward. Return your head to the neutral position. Repeat the exercise, balancing on the other leg.

AVOID
▸ Losing the alignment of your head and back
▸ Raising your shoulders

EFFECTS
▸ Better posture
▸ Better balance
▸ Activation and strengthening of the deep muscles of the spinal column, the core muscles and the lower and upper limbs

DURATION
▸ 5 repetitions in each direction, on each leg

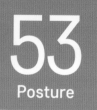

Relaxation of the lateral muscles
▶ for all

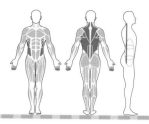

This exercise activates the lateral muscles of the back. It has a relaxing effect on them when they are tense and a stimulating effect on them when they are dormant. To do the movement effectively, sway from side to side in a rhythmic fashion without making a big effort. It has the same principle as the Tail Wag exercise (page 136), but in a sitting position.

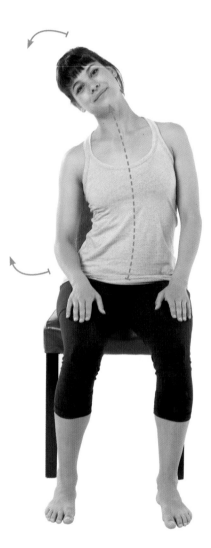

Initial Position

Sitting on the buttocks, with the back straight, without leaning against a backrest.

Action

Tilt your trunk while bringing your buttock and your ear on the same side closer together. Alternate in an energetic fashion from one side to the other.

AVOID	EFFECTS	DURATION
▶ Movement that is too slow or too forced	▶ Relaxation and activation of the lateral muscles ▶ Better posture ▶ Back pain relief	▶ 15 to 30 seconds

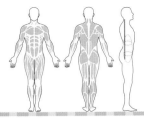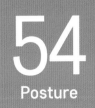
The idea behind this exercise is to sway gently, in rotation, moving the entire spinal column starting from the top. Ideal for relaxing and re-centering the back, this exercise goes well with the previous one, which relaxes the lateral muscles. It is very good for people who work long hours sitting down.

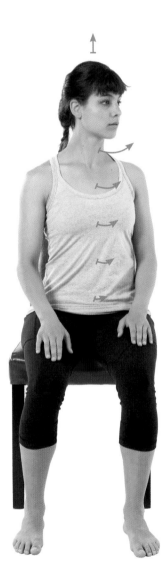

Initial Position
Sitting firmly on the buttocks with the back straight, without leaning against a backrest.

Action
Turn your head slightly to one side and then to the other (about 30 degrees) without making an effort. Relax your body so the movement extends through your entire spinal column.

The Key To Succeed
Allow the swaying to extend through your entire spinal column while keeping it elongated.

AVOID	EFFECTS	DURATION
▸ Losing the elongation of your spinal column	▸ Relaxation and activation of the deep muscles of the back ▸ Better posture	▸ 15 to 30 seconds

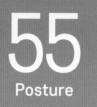

Slump/Straighten up
▶ for all

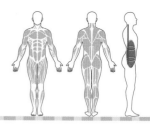

The objective of this exercise is to make us aware of when we are slumped. By going from the slumped (bad) posture to the erect (good) posture, we awaken the postural muscles, become aware of the negative effects of slumping on our body and lose the desire to slouch.

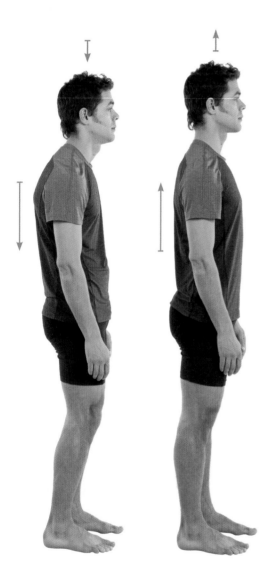

Slump

Initial Position

Standing.

Action

As you exhale, slump by relaxing your back muscles, as though you are extremely tired and the energy is draining from your body.

Straighten Up

Action

As you inhale, straighten up and elongate your spinal column, starting at your head, as though the energy is returning to your body and making you feel stronger and more motivated.

Always end this exercise in the upright position.

The Key To Succeed

Straighten up without effort, using the principles of elongating the spinal column.

AVOID	EFFECTS	DURATION
▶ Straining to stand straight	▶ Renewed awareness of one's posture ▶ Activation of the postural muscles ▶ Better posture	▶ 5 to 10 repetitions

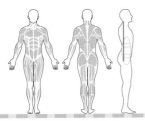
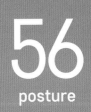
This visualization exercise is especially for kinesthetic types (people who have well-developed body awareness). For others, it will be virtually impossible to do. If this exercise suits you, it will take you on an amazing voyage into your spinal column and to areas that are still unknown.

Visualization does not reside uniquely in the imagination. Just by picturing your head sinking between your shoulders, your muscles and joints start to make tiny adjustments without your having to think about them. Now visualize that your head is light and being pulled toward the ceiling. Doesn't that feel better now?

Compression

Initial Position

Sitting or standing

Action

Imagine that your skull is gently pressing down on your first cervical vertebra. They form a block that is gently pressing down on the second cervical vertebra, which forms a new block, and so on, right down to your sacrum. Do this one vertebra at a time, for a total of 24 vertebrae.

Elongation

Action

Imagine that your skull is slowly disengaging from your first cervical vertebra, which then disengages from the second cervical vertebra, and that the second is disengaging from the third, and so on, down to the sacrum. Elongate your spinal column one vertebra at a time.

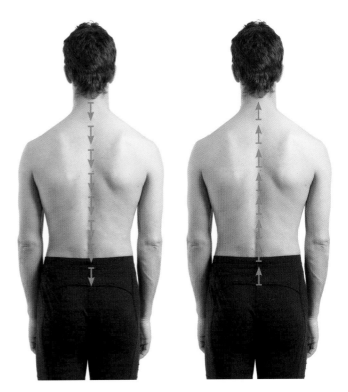

AVOID	EFFECTS	DURATION
▸ Rounding your back	▸ Greater awareness of your spinal column ▸ Better posture	▸ 2 to 5 minutes (with practice, you will be able to do the exercise in less time)

Strengthening

When it comes to muscle strengthening, it is essential to target the deep muscles before working on the superficial muscles. The strengthening exercises that you will find in this section mainly target the core muscles, followed by the deep muscles of the spinal column, which are exercised in a more specific fashion in the postural exercises.

The Key To Succeed

The key words are "fluidity," "control" and "alignment." Fluidity is achieved in movements that demonstrate an efficient use of energy as well as ease. Control requires precise gestures and selecting the right muscles. Alignment refers to good posture and perfect alignment of the different segments of the body. You will learn to master the following elements:

- grounding;
- elongation;
- breathing during exercise;
- relaxation of the muscles that do not need to work (including those of the jaw, face and shoulders);
- activation of the core muscles (we will see how in the following pages).

Repetitions and Series

At what point should you stop? It's simple — you should stop when you can no longer move with fluidity, control and proper alignment. Ideally, you should be able to do these exercises 10 to 30 times. For better results, you can do two series. Doing three series or more is not recommended, given that all of these exercises target the core muscles. It is better to vary the exercises by adding different ones rather than adding more series of the same exercise.

Caution

Strengthening exercises should not be accompanied by pain during or after. They are not recommended if you have acute pain.

57
Strengthening

Half bridge
▸ for all

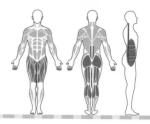

We could have categorized this as a mobility exercise, as the return down to the initial position, one vertebra at a time, is good for the back. The Half Bridge is an essential and complete strengthening exercise that is very effective.

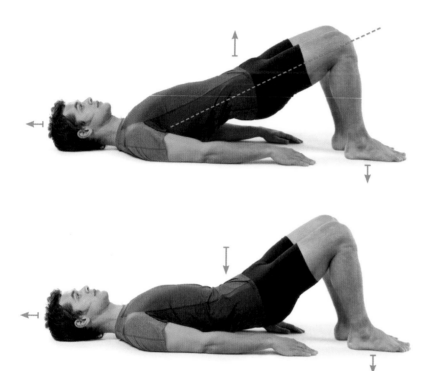

Pelvic Lift

Initial Position

Lying on the back, knees bent and feet aligned with the hips.

Action

As you exhale, lift your pelvis while pushing down equally on both feet.

As you inhale, maintain the position (knees, hips and shoulders aligned).

Pelvic Drop

Action

As you exhale, descend one vertebra at a time, as though you are gluing your back to the floor, from the top to the bottom of your spine. The key is to contract your core muscles by bringing your pubic bone toward your navel during the entire descent.

Inhale in the resting position and then start again.

Tip

Some people may sense that an area in their back feels rigid and does not unroll as smoothly as other areas. This is typical if there is a section of the spinal column (one or more vertebrae) that is not sufficiently mobile. In this case, it is better to focus on mobility exercises and on stretching the lumbar spinal muscles.

If there is no improvement, it is recommended that you consult a health-care professional who will evaluate the condition of your spinal column.

AVOID	EFFECTS	DURATION
▸ Lifting your pelvis too high or not enough ▸ Descending without unrolling the spinal column	▸ Strengthening of the spinal muscles and gluteal muscles ▸ Greater control of the deep muscles of the back	▸ 10 repetitions

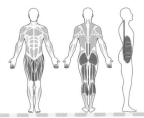

This more advanced version of the Half Bridge calls for greater control and muscle power. It is an excellent way to stabilize the sacroiliac joints. The normal half bridge should be mastered before you move on to this version. This exercise is recommended for runners and people who do a lot of walking.

Pelvic Lift

Initial Position

Lying on the back, knees bent and feet aligned with the hips.

Action

As you exhale, lift your pelvis while pushing down equally on both feet.

As you inhale, maintain the position (knees, hips and shoulders aligned) and extend one leg, keeping both knees at the same height.

Pelvic Drop

Action

As you exhale, descend one vertebra at a time, as if you are gluing your back to the floor, from the top to the bottom of your spine. The key is to contract your core muscles by bringing your pubic bone toward your navel during the entire descent.

Once your pelvis reaches the floor, lower your raised foot to the floor.

Inhale in the resting position, then repeat the exercise with the opposite leg.

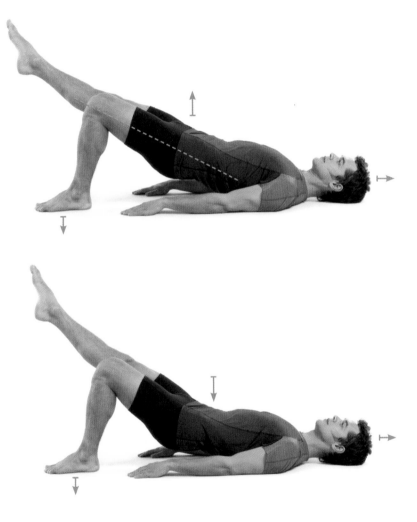

AVOID	EFFECTS	DURATION
▸ Losing the alignment of your pelvis and thighs	▸ Strengthening of the spinal muscles and gluteal muscles ▸ Greater control of the deep muscles of the back ▸ Stabilization of the sacroiliac joints	▸ 5 to 10 repetitions on each side

59

Strengthening

Leg circles
▶ for all

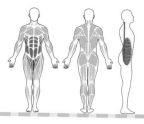

This classic Pilates exercise helps to develop stability in the pelvis and core through the hip movements. It is a good example of a balance posture with stability and mobility.

There is a version of this exercise with the leg extended that is traditionally used in Pilates, but it requires a good deal of flexibility in the hamstring muscles and a lot of power in the psoas muscle. It is not recommended for most people. Attempt it only if you are at an advanced level and if this movement is useful for you (as a dancer, acrobat or athlete, for example).

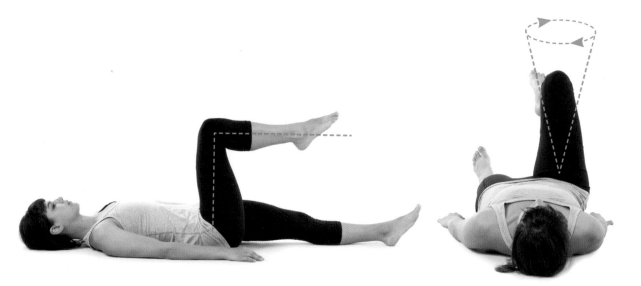

Initial Position

Lying on the back, the knee bent at a 90-degree angle above the hip, the thigh vertical.

Place your hands on either side of your pelvis (anterior superior iliac spine) for greater stability and focus on the movement.

Action

Trace a circle above your hip with your knee. Imagine a cone with the widest part at the top and the narrowest part just above the hip.

As you inhale, turn your knee outward.

As you exhale, turn your knee inward.

The Key To Succeed

Always keep your pelvis level and do not let it rock from side to side.

AVOID

▶ Raising your pelvis
▶ Making circles of different sizes or irregular shapes

EFFECTS

▶ Greater stability of the pelvis, lower back and hips
▶ Greater control of the core muscles

DURATION

▶ 5 repetitions in each direction, on each side

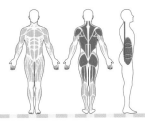

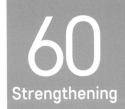

A basic, risk-free exercise to improve stability in the back and to prepare it for a more difficult standing exercise.

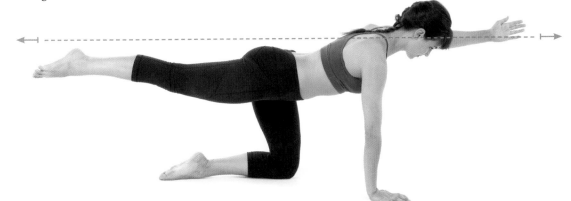

Table

Initial Position

On all fours, knees under the hips, hands under the shoulders and the spinal column straight and long.

Visualization

Imagine a thread running from the tip of your coccyx (tailbone) to the wall behind you, and a thread running from the top of your skull to the wall in front of you.

Visualize your spinal column lengthening.

Action

As you exhale, extend your leg directly behind you. At the same time, extend the opposite arm directly in front of you, palm turned inward. As you inhale, return to the initial position. Repeat this exercise on the opposite side.

The Key To Succeed

Be sure to activate your core muscles during this exercise.

Tip

If the balancing table is difficult to do, start by only lifting your leg, and then only your arm. Once you have mastered these versions, you will be ready to raise your arm and leg at the same time.

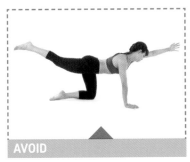

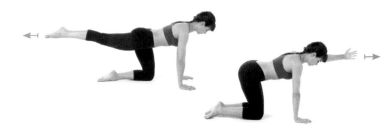

AVOID

▸ Losing your alignment

EFFECTS

▸ Strengthening of the core muscles and back muscles
▸ Greater control of the deep muscles of back
▸ Greater stability

DURATION

▸ 10 repetitions on each side

61
Strengthening

Balancing table with diagonals
▶ intermediate to advanced

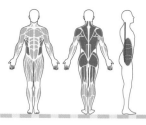

This version of the Balancing Table activates the back muscles more than the previous exercise because of the additional activation of the lateral muscles. This makes it a more comprehensive exercise.

Initial Position

On all fours, knees under the hips, hands under the shoulders and the spinal column straight and long.

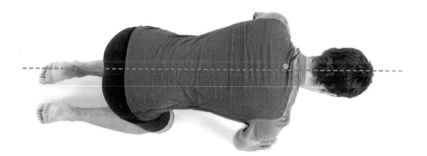

Exhaling

Action

1. Do the Balancing Table exercise (60). Extend your right leg, pushing your heel backward until your leg is slightly horizontal. At the same time, extend your left arm slightly horizontally, your palm turned inward.

Inhaling

Action

2. Open your extended arm and leg about 30 degrees to form a diagonal line.

Exhaling

Action

3. Return to Step 1 (Balancing Table).

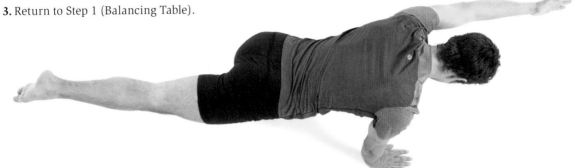

Inhaling

Action

4. Return to the initial position. On all fours, knees under the hips, hands under the shoulders and the spinal column straight and long. Repeat this exercise on the opposite side.

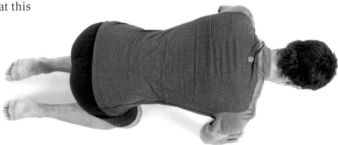

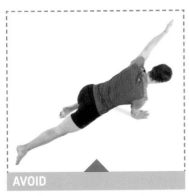

Note
Alternate sides with each repetition.

The Key To Succeed
Keep your spinal column aligned and elongated.

AVOID

▸ Losing your alignment

EFFECTS

▸ Strengthening of the core muscles and back muscles
▸ Greater control of the deep muscles of the back
▸ Greater stability

DURATION

▸ 5 repetitions on each side

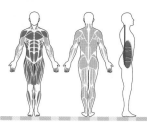

This exercise is labeled as isometric contractions (without movement) because it holds a position to build strength without movement in the joint or muscle. It mainly activates the anterior chain (abdominal and pectoral muscles). People often do the plank incorrectly, putting their back at risk. But when done properly, it activates the deep muscles and is one of the best stabilization exercises. It is recommended that you fully master the Half Plank before you do the full Plank.

   This exercise is not recommended for those with a herniated disk. People who suffer from high blood pressure should hold this posture for no more than 10 seconds.

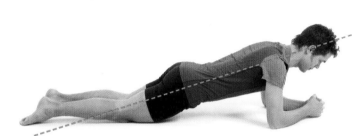

Half Plank

Initial Position

Facing the floor, resting on the knees, hands joined together and the elbows apart to form a tripod.

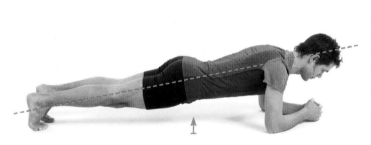

Plank

Action

For both the Half Plank and Plank, start by sliding your scapulae (shoulder blades) toward your pelvis, then elongate your spinal column, activate your core muscles (pelvic floor, transversus abdominis and abdominals) and push your elbows into the floor (and your toes into the ground for plank). Lift your pelvis and assume the Half Plank or Plank position. Hold this position and breathe.

The Key To Succeed

Keep your core muscles contracted and your spinal column elongated.
   Do not arch your back.

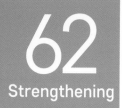

AVOID
▸ Arching your back and raising your shoulders

EFFECTS
▸ Strengthening of the core muscles
▸ Greater stability

DURATION
▸ 5 to 60 seconds (increase the duration very gradually, without going to the maximum the first few times

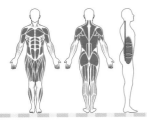

The Side Plank, which is complementary to the previous plank, is even more difficult to master. It activates the lateral muscles (large dorsal, quadratus lumborum, obliques, lateral spinal flexors) in a significant fashion. This exercise requires a great degree of control, and it is recommended that you master it before you increase the duration, doing several short repetitions instead of a long one. Be sure to master the Half Plank before moving on to the full Plank.

   This exercise is not recommended if you have a herniated disk. People who suffer from high blood pressure should do this for no more than 10 seconds.

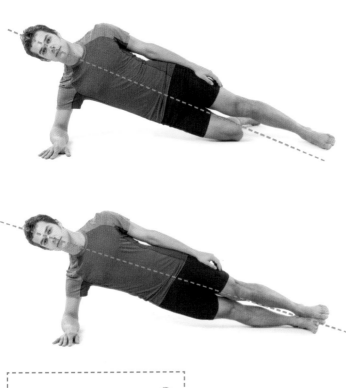

Half Side Plank

Initial Position

Lying on the side, the elbow under the shoulder.

Side Plank

Action

For both the Half Plank and Plank, start by lying on one side, lining up the elbow with the scapulae (shoulder blade) to form a 90-degree angle, then elongate your spinal column and activate your core muscles (pelvic floor, transversus abdominis and abdominals).

   For the Half Plank, bend the knee of the leg touching the floor. Push your elbow into the floor, (and lift your pelvis to assume the Half Plank or Plank position. Hold this position and breathe. Repeat the exercise on the opposite side.

The Key To Succeed

Keep your core muscles contracted and your spinal column elongated.

   At no time should your back bend toward the floor.

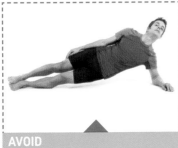

AVOID	EFFECTS	DURATION
▸ Bending your back ▸ Raising your shoulder	▸ Strengthening of the lateral muscles and core muscles ▸ Greater stability	▸ 5 to 60 seconds (increase the duration very gradually, without going to the maximum the first few times) on each side

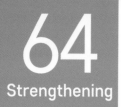

Rotary plank on wall
▶ intermediate to advanced

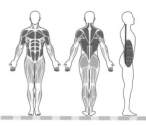

This exercise is excellent for training the back muscles at the same time as the abdominal muscles. All you need is a wall and a desire to have more control over your body movements.

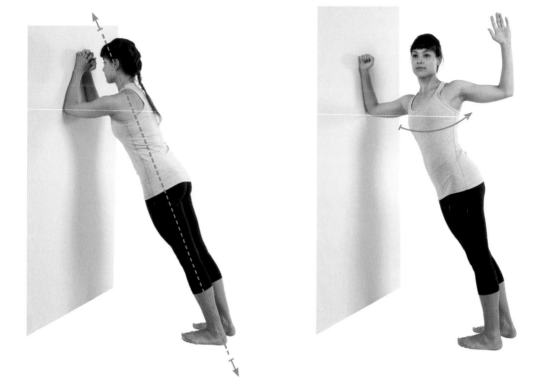

Initial Position

In the Plank position, leaning against a wall at an angle of about 30 degrees (15 degrees to make the exercise easier), your hands joined and your elbows spread apart, your core muscles contracted and your spinal column elongated.

Action

As you inhale, turn your trunk as if to look to the side, bringing one elbow back. As you exhale, return to the center. Repeat the exercise on the opposite side.

The Key To Succeed

Activate your core muscles and keep your spinal column elongated throughout the exercise.

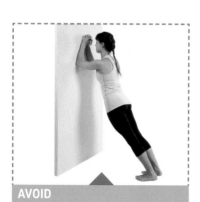

AVOID	EFFECTS	DURATION
▶ Arching your back	▶ Strengthening of the back and core muscles	▶ 5 to 10 repetitions on each side

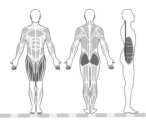

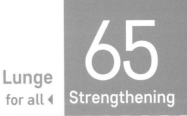

The Lunge is an excellent exercise for activating the back and lower limbs. The key is to keep your pelvis aligned and your spinal column elongated. This exercise has the added advantage of stimulating the proprioceptors. The Lunge is also transferable to everyday movement and a number of different sports.

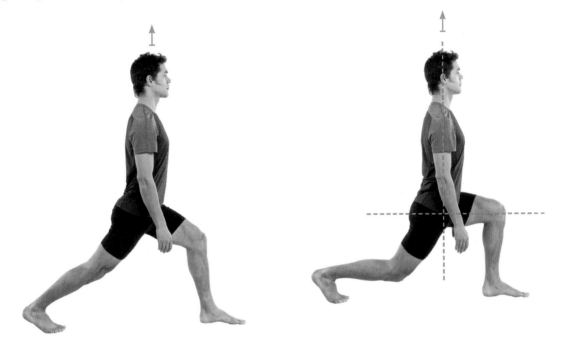

Initial Position

Standing, the feet aligned with the hips. One foot is ahead of the other (about 12 inches/30 cm) farther than a normal step). The pelvis is level and the pubic bone faces forward.

Action

As you inhale, lower yourself in a straight line until your thigh is horizontal without allowing your knee to extend over your foot. Keep your back straight, as though a thread were pulling the top of your head upward. Rise in a straight line as you exhale. Repeat the exercise on the opposite side.

The Key To Succeed

Your pelvis should remain horizontal (without turning or tilting) throughout the exercise.

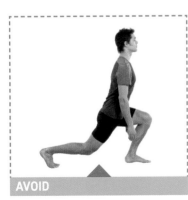

AVOID

▸ Bending your trunk
▸ Allowing your knee to jut out past your foot

EFFECTS

▸ Strengthening of the legs and the deep muscles of the back
▸ Better posture

DURATION

▸ 5 to 10 repetitions on each side

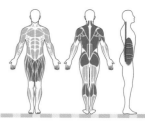

Derived from a yoga posture, the diagonal exercise helps to strengthen the deep and superficial muscles of the back while disengaging the ankles. The challenge is to stretch the hamstring thoroughly while maintaining the position. This exercise protects your back and prepares it for activities that require bending while keeping your back straight.

Initial Position

Standing, one foot in front of the other (with a fair distance between the feet, as in the Lunge). The feet are aligned with the hips and the arms are raised toward the ceiling, palms turned inward.

Action

Move your trunk forward, extend your arms until you feel a pull in your hamstring and form a straight line. Repeat the exercise on the opposite side.

Visualization

Imagine that a straight line is running through your body, from your back heel to your fingertips.

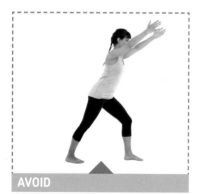

AVOID	EFFECTS	DURATION
▶ Losing your alignment	▶ Strengthening of the deep and superficial muscles of the back ▶ Increased suppleness in the ankles ▶ Greater stability	▶ 15 to 30 seconds on each side

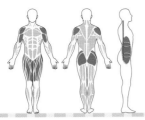

A classic exercise, the Squat is a useful basic posture for many everyday actions. It is a very effective exercise for strengthening the thighs and gluteal muscles. When done correctly, the Squat also helps to activate the postural muscles. It is important to keep your spinal column elongated.

Initial Position

Standing, the feet spread a little farther than the width of the hips. The arms are raised to shoulder height and the palms are turned inward. The feet must be firmly planted on the floor before doing this exercise.

Action

As you inhale, bend your knees at a 90-degree angle, keeping your spinal column straight and elongated. Keep your shoulders down and extend your arms forward all the way to your fingertips.

As you exhale, push down equally on both feet and return to the initial position.

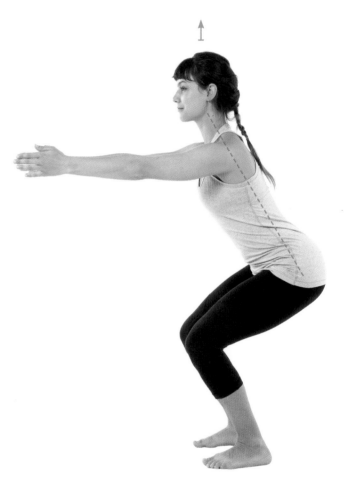

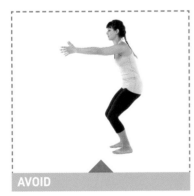

AVOID

▸ Rounding your back

EFFECTS

▸ Strengthening of the thighs and gluteal muscles
▸ Strengthening of the core and back muscles

DURATION

▸ 10 to 15 repetitions

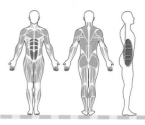

The Half Roll-up helps work the abdominals by activating the back in a significant fashion. The number of repetitions is not important — it is the way you do the exercise that matters. Use all the layers of the abdominals (superficial and deep) as well the pelvic floor muscles for more tangible results.

Caution: This exercise should not be accompanied by pain in the back. If you feel discomfort in the back of your neck, try some neck relaxation exercises to alleviate it before continuing this exercise.

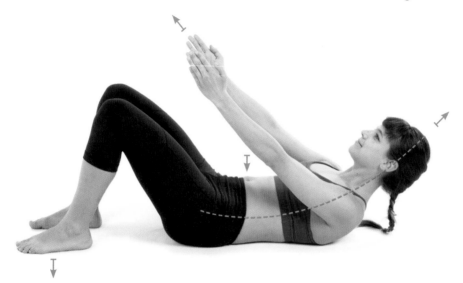

Initial Position

Lying on the back, knees bent and feet aligned with the hips, arms raised to a 45-degree angle, palms turned inward, the back of the neck and the spinal column elongated and the scapulae (shoulder blades) pulled toward the pelvis.

Action

As you exhale, start by bringing your pubic bone toward your navel, contracting your pelvic floor muscles and bringing your navel toward your spinal column.

Next, lengthen the back of your neck by bending your head down toward your neck. Raise your trunk until your scapulae (shoulder blades) lift off the floor, without going farther. Extend your arms all the way to your fingertips and keep them parallel.

As you inhale, return to the initial position.

The Key To Succeed

Activate your core muscles while keeping your spinal column elongated.

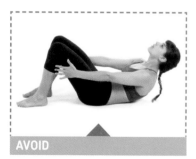

AVOID	EFFECTS	DURATION
▸ Pulling up too high ▸ Raising your shoulders ▸ Neglecting to contract your pelvic floor muscles	▸ Strengthening of the abdominal muscles and the core muscles	▸ 10 repetitions

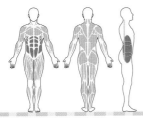

This alternative to the Half Roll-up targets the oblique muscles. The deep muscles of the back are activated to control the movement. The advantage of this exercise is that your parallel arms help to maintain your central alignment as you perform the twisting movements with your trunk.

The action is the same as for the Half Roll-up with the addition of one arm moving ahead of the other to twist the trunk. In the photo below, both arms are raised but the left arm is farther ahead, which pulls the trunk to the right.

This exercise should not cause back pain. If you feel discomfort in the back of your neck, try some neck relaxation exercises to alleviate it before continuing this exercise.

Initial Position

Lying on the back, knees bent and feet aligned with the hips.

Action

As you exhale, rise and move one arm ahead of the other. As you inhale, descend while bringing your arm back to the original position. Change arms with each repetition.

The Key To Succeed

Keep your arms parallel while sliding your scapulae (shoulder blades) toward your pelvis.

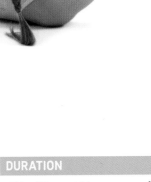

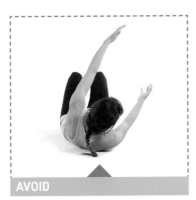

AVOID	**EFFECTS**	**DURATION**
▸ Losing the alignment in your arms	▸ Strengthening of the abdominal, oblique and core muscles	▸ 5 to 10 repetitions on each side

70
Strengthening

Ultimate pelvic floor contraction
▶ intermediate to advanced

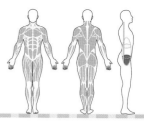

Once you have mastered the pelvic floor contraction, have fun doing the following versions. Your pelvic floor muscles will be put to the challenge, but your pelvis and back will greatly benefit. For women and men, this exercise activates the reproductive system. These contractions are ideal during pregnancy and for recovery after childbirth.

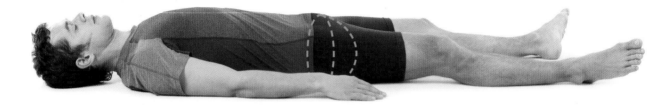

Initial Position
Lying on the back or standing.

Action
1. As you exhale, contract your pelvic floor muscles. As you inhale, relax the muscles halfway, then completely. **Duration:** 10 repetitions
2. As you exhale, contract your pelvic floor halfway, then completely. As you inhale, gradually relax. **Duration:** 10 repetitions

3. Contract and release your pelvic floor muscles as quickly as possible for 20 seconds. Over time, you will increase both your speed and endurance. **Duration:** 3 repetitions (you can go up to 10)
4. Contract your pelvic floor muscles as much as possible and hold the contraction for 3 breaths. Over time, this will improve both the quality of the contraction as well as your endurance. **Duration:** 3 to 5 repetitions

AVOID	EFFECTS	DURATION
▶ Contracting your superficial gluteal muscles	▶ Improved contraction and relaxation of the pelvic floor muscles	▶ See duration times for each action

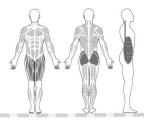

This exercise reconditions and rebalances the pelvic muscles, which may be imbalanced if you have a misaligned pelvis or you do assymetrical activities, such as canoeing or racquet sports. The objective is to stabilize the base of your spinal column. Think of it as creating a solid foundation that will eventually support a building. If your pelvis is misaligned, you need to do this exercise for at least two weeks in order to obtain long-lasting results.

Activating all the muscles attached to the pelvis at the same time in a well-aligned movement helps to restore balance.

If you are unable to do the movement symmetrically, even with practice, it is possible that your pelvis is misaligned or that you have one leg longer than the other. Consult a health-care professional for confirmation.

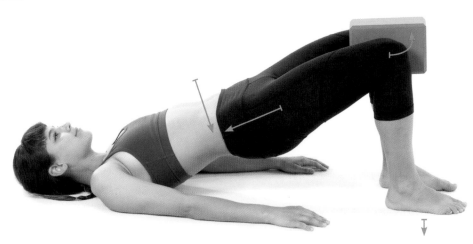

Initial Position

Lying on the back, knees bent and feet aligned with the hips, with a cushion or a ball between the knees. Arms are next to the body, palms on the floor.

Action

As you exhale, press the cushion or ball between your knees, contract your pelvic floor and your transversus abdominis. Lift your pelvis while pushing down equally on both feet.

As you inhale, hold your position, keeping your pelvis level.

As you exhale, lower your pelvis one vertebra at a time, from top to bottom, while continuing to contract your pelvic floor, transversus abdominis and adductors (maintaining the pressure on the cushion or ball).

As you inhale, return to the starting position.

AVOID
▸ Pressing your knees together too tightly

EFFECTS
▸ Rebalancing of the pelvis

DURATION
▸ 10 repetitions

Balance

Muscle contraction is controlled by the nervous system. Starting at the brain, passing through the spinal cord and the nerves, the nervous system sends information to the muscles and, in turn, receives information about the muscles. The nervous system and the muscular system are thus interrelated, which explains why stress or pain causes muscle tension. In order for your muscles to be relaxed, your nervous system needs to be relaxed. These balance exercises are designed with this in mind.

The Key To Succeed

During these exercises, the first thing to do is focus on your breathing.

Duration

Two minutes is all it takes to make a difference. If the exercise makes you feel good, you can do it as long as you like.

Caution

As with the breathing exercises, these may be difficult for some people. If you are not experiencing pain or fatigue but are chronically stressed, it may be better to do some cardio exercises to help you expend excess energy before attempting these exercises.

Derived from the principles of alternative medicine, this technique is an effective way to restore balance when you feel scattered, in pain or under stress. The hands are placed on the body's most important centers responsible for helping to restore balance.

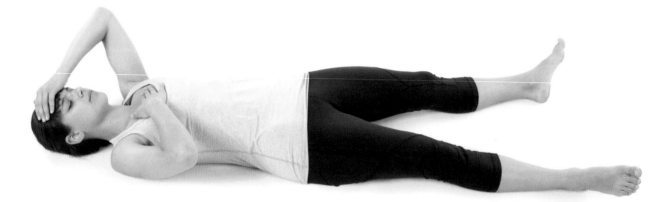

Head-Heart Balance

Initial Position

Lying on the back, one hand placed flat on the forehead, the other flat in the middle of the sternum.

Action

Breathe slowly and deeply, keeping your hands relaxed, for 1 minute.

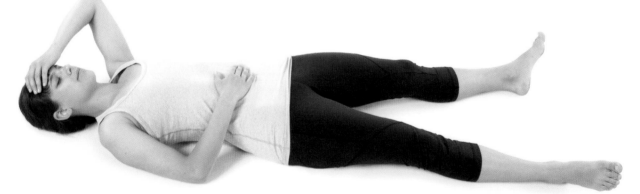

Head-Abdomen Balance

Initial Position

Lying on the back, one hand placed flat on the forehead, the other flat on the navel.

Action

Breathe slowly and deeply, keeping your hands relaxed, for 1 minute.

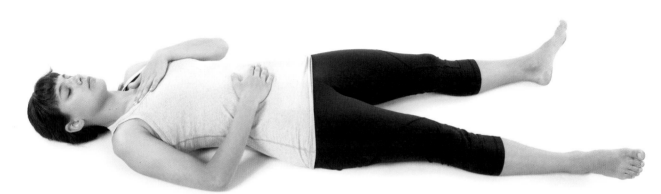

Abdomen-Heart Balance

Initial Position

Lying on the back, one hand placed flat in the middle of the sternum, the other flat on the navel.

Action

Breathe slowly and deeply, keeping your hands relaxed, for 1 minute.

The Key To Succeed

It is important to let your body relax while you breathe calmly.

Visualization

Visualize that the areas underneath your hands are relaxing and that the circulation between them is improving.

AVOID	EFFECTS	DURATION
▸ Pressing with your hands	▸ Better posture ▸ More efficient breathing ▸ Back pain relief	▸ 3 to 5 minutes total

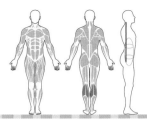

Imagine you are lying in a sleeping car on a train and rocking back and forth to the rhythm of the locomotive. This exercise may not take you on a voyage, but it does serve two purposes. First, it relaxes the spinal column, from the head to the sacrum. Second, it helps rebalance the nervous system. Have fun accelerating gradually and see how you feel afterward. Then, do the reverse, gradually slowing down. In time, you will find the ideal rhythm to help restore your balance.

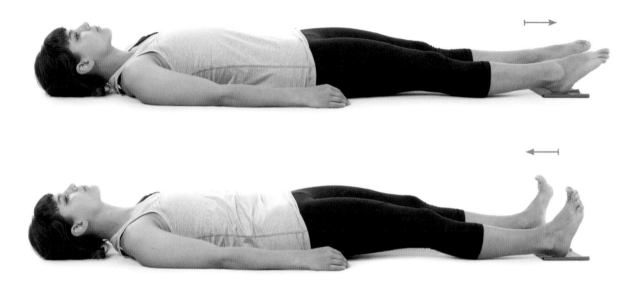

Initial Position
Lying on the back, knees slightly bent, heels placed on an anti-slip surface (an exercise mat is ideal) to help facilitate the rocking motion.

Action
Make your entire body rock by moving only your ankles and feet. Point your feet forward and pull them back in an energetic fashion, without straining, and while remaining relaxed.

AVOID
▶ Letting your heels slide on the floor

EFFECTS
▶ Restored balance in the nervous system
▶ Greater mobility in the spinal column
▶ Back pain relief

DURATION
▶ 30 to 60 seconds (about 140 back-and-forth movements a minute)

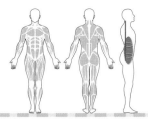

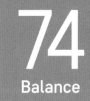

Do this exercise to reconnect your central axis and center yourself. It is amazingly effective for restoring energy and improving posture. It activates the extremities of the central axis, including the center of the pelvic floor and the top of the skull (also called the vertex) along with the core muscles.

Initial Position
Standing.

Action
1. Pull in the center of your pelvic floor.
2. With the tip of your tongue, apply pressure to the roof of your mouth, toward the top of your skull.
3. Pull in your navel toward the middle of your abdomen. Once these three elements are activated, maintain them by visualizing your central axis.

Visualization
Imagine a laser beam is passing through your body, from the top of your skull to the middle of your pelvic floor.

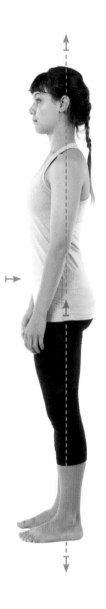

AVOID	EFFECTS	DURATION
▸ Relaxing one element and activating the others	▸ Better posture ▸ Feeling centered	▸ 15 to 60 seconds

Back-relief position
▶ for all

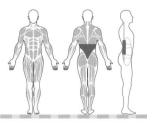

This position is the first one you should adopt to relax your back. Adapt it so that you are comfortable, which will help your nervous system to relax. It is derived from a technique invented by American osteopath Dr. Lawrence H. Jones.

The idea is to make your nervous system dormant by helping it forget that your muscles are tense. By slowly returning to the normal position, you trick your nervous system, which forgets the initial state of tension.

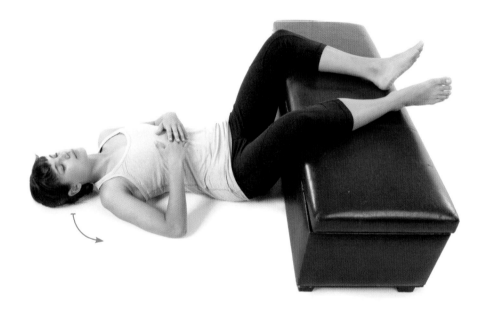

Initial Position

Lying on the back in front of a bed or sofa, legs positioned so that the knees and hips are bent about 90 degrees. Place a pillow under your head for more comfort.

If you have more pain on one side of your body than the other, bend your trunk and head slightly to the side that hurts more.

Action

Maintain the position for a minimum of 2 minutes, then relax slowly and lie on your side before getting up.

The Key To Succeed

Find the most comfortable position, in which you have the least pain, without modifying the position too much.

AVOID
▶ Remaining in a position that is not comfortable

EFFECTS
▶ Relief of lower back pain

DURATION
▶ 2 to 15 minutes

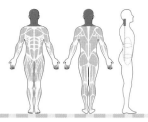
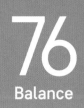
How do you release the tension that has accumulated in your temporal muscles (temples) and your neck in just 15 seconds? Here is a very soothing exercise that I developed when I was spending an inordinate amount of time at the computer. It has helped many people since then who make it part of their daily routine.

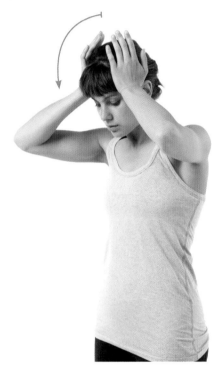

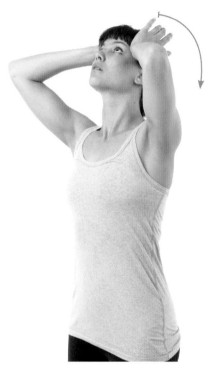

Initial Position

Sitting or standing, the palms of the hands resting on the temples.

Action

Lightly press your hands together (to get into the temporal muscles) and push your palms upward (to stretch the muscles).

Maintaining the pressure with your hands, slowly bend your head forward and then tilt it backward.

The Key To Succeed

Adjust the pressure in the palms of your hands so that you are pulling the temporal muscles upward without compressing your temples.

AVOID	EFFECTS	DURATION
▸ Pressing too hard on your temples	▸ Relief for the temples, jaw, head and neck	▸ 3 to 5 repetitions

Shoulders and neck relaxation
▸ for all

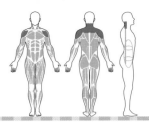

Do you ever have the feeling that your shoulders are attached to your ears? If so, this exercise will help relax your neck, bring your shoulders down and lengthen the back of your neck.

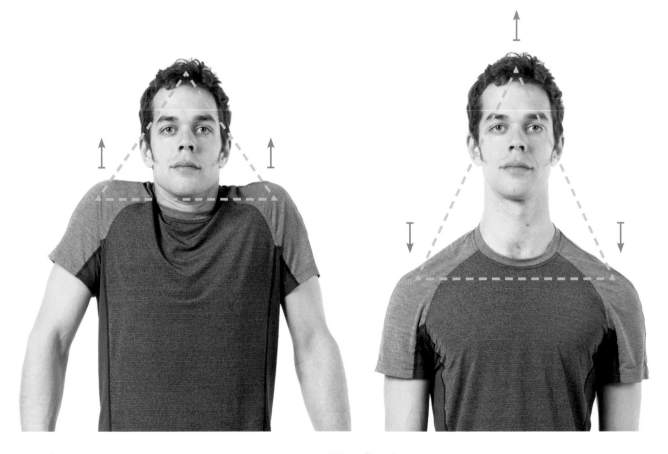

Action
As you inhale, raise your shoulders toward your ears. As you exhale, relax them gradually and completely, keeping your neck relaxed.

Visualization
Imagine your skull and shoulders as a triangle with three points, the top of your skull being at the top. Try to make the triangle smaller by raising your shoulders, then larger by lowering them.

AVOID
▸ Straining to raise your shoulders

EFFECTS
▸ Relief of tension in the neck and shoulders

DURATION
▸ 5 repetitions

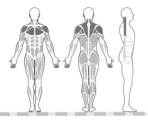
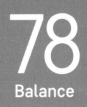
This exercise is a very simple and effective way to release tension accumulated in the chest, shoulders and neck. You can do this in combination with the previous exercise.

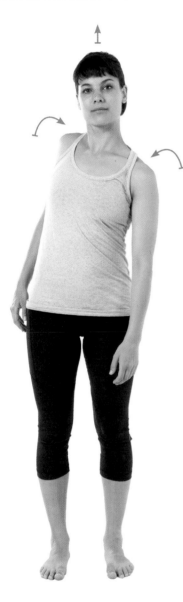

Initial Position
Standing or sitting (but without letting the back touch the chair's backrest).

Action
Turn one shoulder back while keeping the other one facing forward, and then turn back the other shoulder.

The Key To Succeed
A fluid, effortless movement, keeping the jaw relaxed.

AVOID
▸ Raising your shoulder too high

EFFECTS
▸ Relief of tension in the chest (especially the area between the scapulae), neck and shoulders
▸ More efficient breathing

DURATION
▸ 10 repetitions on each side

Overall back relaxation
▶ for all

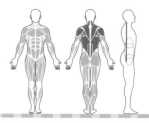

I highly recommend this exercise if you are looking for a quick and easy way to relax your back. The pelvis and leg movements are slightly reminiscent of the Twist dance move, so you may want to do it behind closed doors.

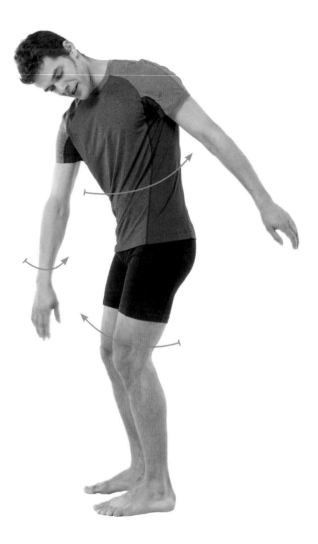

Initial Position
Standing, knees slightly bent, neck relaxed and head falling slightly forward.

Visualization
Imagine that your arms are as soft as bread dough.

Action
Swing your arms around, one forward and one backward, letting your back, pelvis and legs move freely as you swing to one side, then the other.

AVOID
▶ Tensing up while moving

EFFECTS
▶ Relief of back tension
▶ More efficient breathing

DURATION
▶ 15 seconds

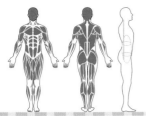

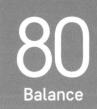

Neuromuscular relaxation is a technique that has been around for years. It is an excellent way to relax the muscular and nervous systems and help relieve chronic or acute pain. It also helps you to become more aware of your body.

This relaxation technique can vary in duration. You may not be able to completely relax certain areas. This is normal. By repeating the exercise, your ability to relax will increase.

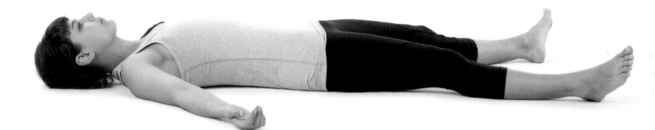

Initial Position
Lying on the back.

Action
Imagine that each body part listed is becoming heavy and soft:
1. One lower limb after the other (foot, hamstring, knee, thigh, buttocks).
2. Go up the spinal column toward the shoulders (pelvis, lower back, chest, scapulae).
3. One upper limb after the other (shoulder, arms, neck, forearms and hands).
4. Go up to the head (neck, jaw, eyes, forehead, entire head).

AVOID	EFFECTS	DURATION
▸ Trying to go too fast	▸ Muscle relaxation ▸ Restored balance in the nervous system ▸ Relief of back tension ▸ More efficient breathing	▸ 10 to 20 minutes

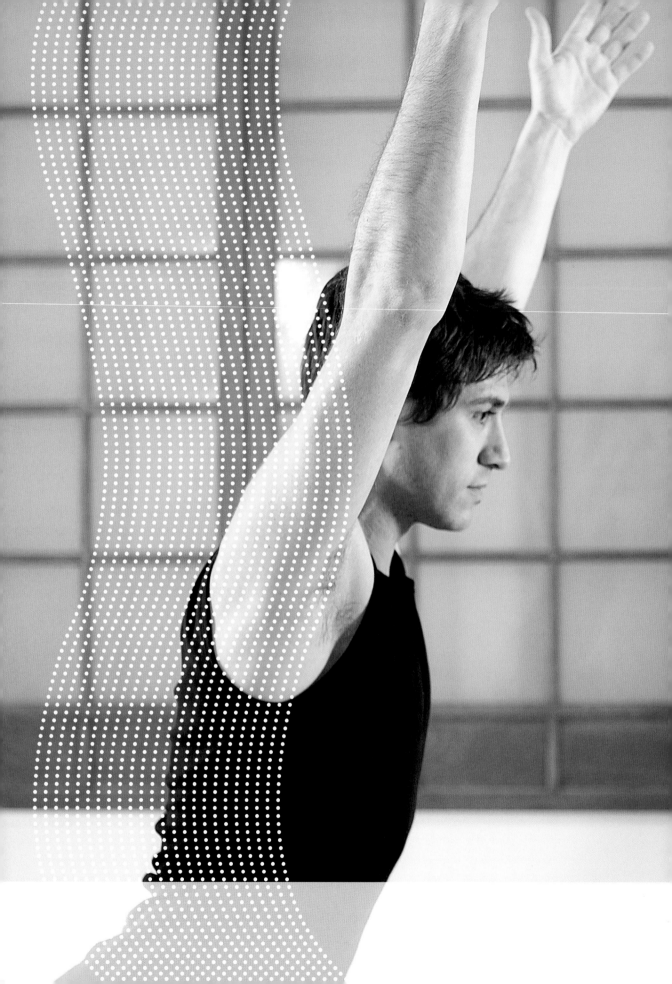

CHAPTER 7: ROUTINES

One, Two, Three, Action

Now you're ready to select the routine or routines that suit you best. You will find quite a few choices here that meet many different needs and offer variety. It would be simple for me to simply say, "Here are the 10 miracle exercises. Do them – they're for everyone!" However, like many things in life, there is no miracle recipe that suits all.

Your choice of routine also depends on how much time you have to devote to it. Many of the routines should be suitable, even if you're short on time. More than 20 of them can be done in 10 minutes or less. After all, what's 10 minutes out of a day to treat your back the way it deserves to be treated?

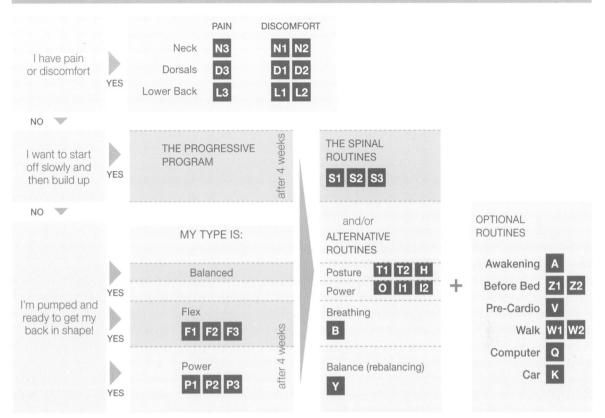

In Case of Pain or Discomfort

Pain

If you are experiencing a lot of back pain, doing or forcing strengthening exercises can increase pain rather than diminish it. The adage, "No pain, no gain" definitely has no place here. No exercise should increase pain during or after. The objective is to help diminish pain before moving on to a more active routine.

Discomfort

Most people live with neck tension, twinges between the shoulder blades and stiffness in the lower back. Everyone has a fragile zone. If you live with back discomfort that is fairly constant, you should do exercises to help release tension by targeting your fragile zone. At the same time, you need to understand that the spinal column functions both as a unit and as a group.

The lumbar muscles work as a team with the dorsal and cervical muscles. Your back is not aware that anatomists have divided it into sections. That is why you will find a common base in every routine that trains the entire back, no matter what zone is being targeted.

The Progressive Program

If you want to follow a program that will help you gradually master each exercise, increasing the level of difficulty one day at a time, the Progressive Program is for you. It only requires 2 minutes a day at the beginning, building up to 15 minutes a day after 4 weeks. This gives you sufficient time to thoroughly understand the basic back exercises and integrate them into your daily routine.

"Balanced," "Flex" or "Power" Type

If you are the "flex" or "power" type (see page 98), it is recommended that you work on your fragile zones before moving on to the basic routines. Spend about 4 weeks focusing on your weaker area. If you are the "balanced" type, you can go directly to the Spinal routine stage.

The Spinal Routines

The exercises in the Spinal Routine were designed to meet the complete needs of your back. They form the heart of your training program. Do a Spinal Routine two to four times a week and your back will see improvement. You can also combine these routines with alternative ones for even more variety.

Alternative Routines

Varying the routine helps you achieve better results in the long term. These routines target specific areas — posture, muscle strength, breathing and rebalancing your nervous system, depending on what other areas you would like to work on.

Routines of the Moment

You can also add any of these routines to your daily routine. When you wake up, before you go to bed, before doing cardio or after a long walk — all good times to do something good for your back. Some exercises can be treated like mini-breaks, for example, to reduce tension if you're working at a computer. Other exercises can be done while driving if you spend a lot of the time on the road.

Sample Program (For a "Power"-Type Person)

Weeks 1 to 4:	▷	Flex routines only
Weeks 5 and 6:	▷	Flex routines and Spinal routines in equal parts
Weeks 7 and 8:	▷	25% Flex routines and 75% Spinal routines
Once you are balanced:	▷	Spinal routines only

List of Routines

For more information about the numbered exercises in this section, see Chapter 6, page 104.

	Name	Duration	Level
S1	Spinal 1	20 minutes	Intermediate
S2	Spinal 2	30 minutes	Intermediate to advanced
S3	Spinal 3	40 minutes	Intermediate to advanced
F1	Flex 1	5 minutes	For all
F2	Flex 2	12 minutes	For all
F3	Flex 3	20 minutes	For all
P1	Power 1	4 minutes	Intermediate
P2	Power 2	8 minutes	Intermediate
P3	Power 3	15 minutes	Intermediate
T1	Posture 1	5 minutes	For all
T2	Posture 2	12 minutes	For all
H	Helical	8 minutes	For all
O	360°	4 minutes per cycle	Intermediate to advanced
A	Awakening	5 minutes	For all
I1	Intense 1	10 minutes	Intermediate
I2	Intense 2	22 minutes	Intermediate to advanced
B	Breathing	12 minutes	For all
Y	Balance	10 minutes	For all
Z1	Before bed 1	3 minutes	For all
Z2	Before bed 2	10 minutes	For all
V	Pre-cardio	5 minutes	For all
W1	After a long walk 1	4 minutes	For all
W2	After a long walk 2	8 minutes	For all
K	Car	—	For all
Q	Computer	—	For all
D1	Dorsal 1	4 minutes	For all
D2	Dorsal 2	12 minutes	For all
D3	Dorsal relief	10 minutes	For all
L1	Lumbar 1	5 minutes	For all
L2	Lumbar 2	18 minutes	For all
L3	Lumbar relief	10 minutes	For all
N1	Neck 1	3 minutes	For all
N2	Neck 2	10 minutes	For all
N3	Neck relief	10 minutes	For all

Spinal 1 / 20 minutes
Excellent time-effectiveness ratio
▶ **Intermediate**
See Chapter 6 for more details on each numbered exercise.

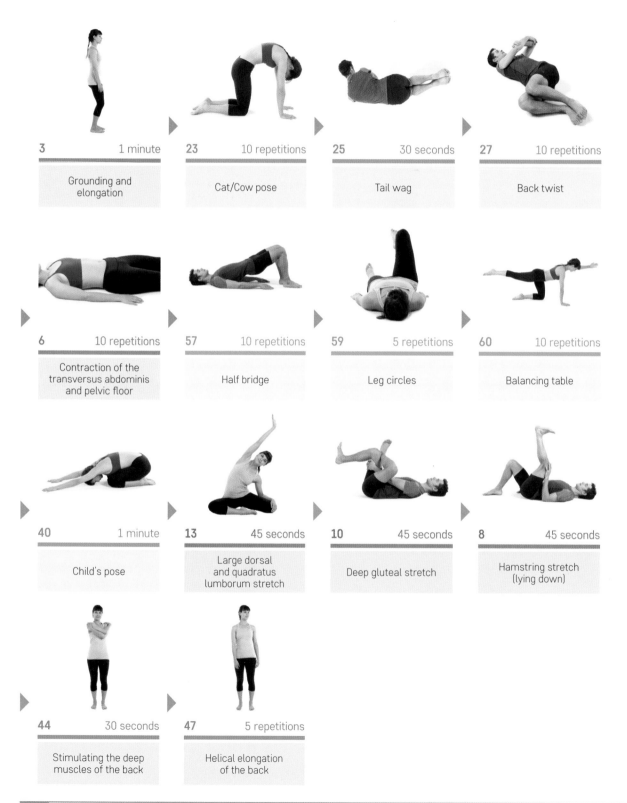

3   1 minute
Grounding and elongation

23   10 repetitions
Cat/Cow pose

25   30 seconds
Tail wag

27   10 repetitions
Back twist

6   10 repetitions
Contraction of the transversus abdominis and pelvic floor

57   10 repetitions
Half bridge

59   5 repetitions
Leg circles

60   10 repetitions
Balancing table

40   1 minute
Child's pose

13   45 seconds
Large dorsal and quadratus lumborum stretch

10   45 seconds
Deep gluteal stretch

8   45 seconds
Hamstring stretch (lying down)

44   30 seconds
Stimulating the deep muscles of the back

47   5 repetitions
Helical elongation of the back

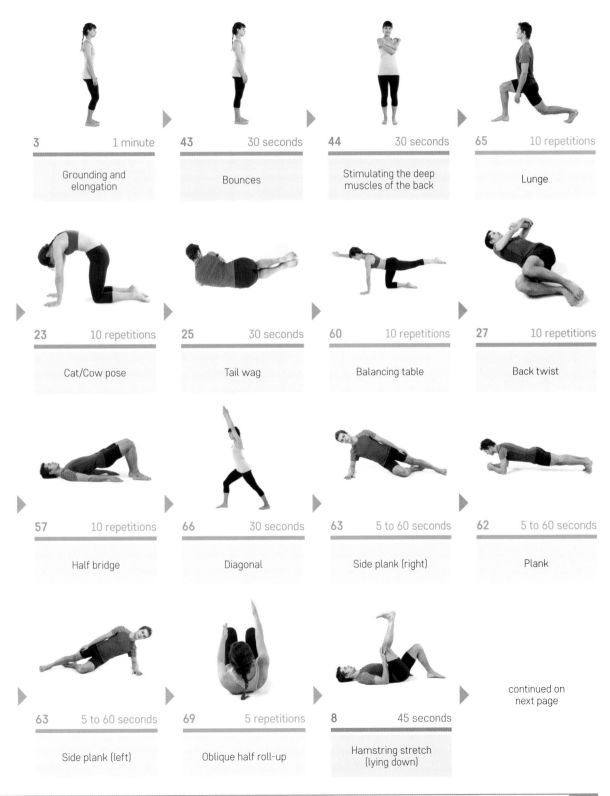

3 1 minute	**43** 30 seconds	**44** 30 seconds	**65** 10 repetitions
Grounding and elongation	Bounces	Stimulating the deep muscles of the back	Lunge

23 10 repetitions	**25** 30 seconds	**60** 10 repetitions	**27** 10 repetitions
Cat/Cow pose	Tail wag	Balancing table	Back twist

57 10 repetitions	**66** 30 seconds	**63** 5 to 60 seconds	**62** 5 to 60 seconds
Half bridge	Diagonal	Side plank (right)	Plank

63 5 to 60 seconds	**69** 5 repetitions	**8** 45 seconds	
Side plank (left)	Oblique half roll-up	Hamstring stretch (lying down)	

continued on next page

Spinal 2 / 30 minutes (continued)
To exercise your entire back in less than 30 minutes
▶ **Intermediate to advanced**
See Chapter 6 for more details on each numbered exercise.

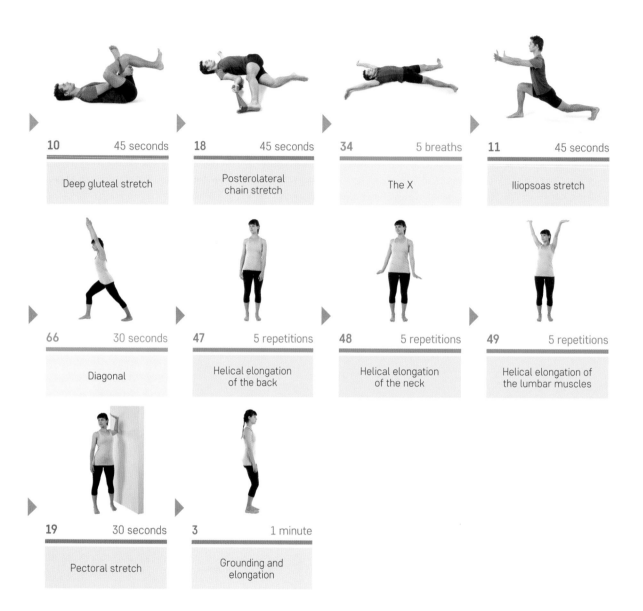

10　　45 seconds

Deep gluteal stretch

18　　45 seconds

Posterolateral chain stretch

34　　5 breaths

The X

11　　45 seconds

Iliopsoas stretch

66　　30 seconds

Diagonal

47　　5 repetitions

Helical elongation of the back

48　　5 repetitions

Helical elongation of the neck

49　　5 repetitions

Helical elongation of the lumbar muscles

19　　30 seconds

Pectoral stretch

3　　1 minute

Grounding and elongation

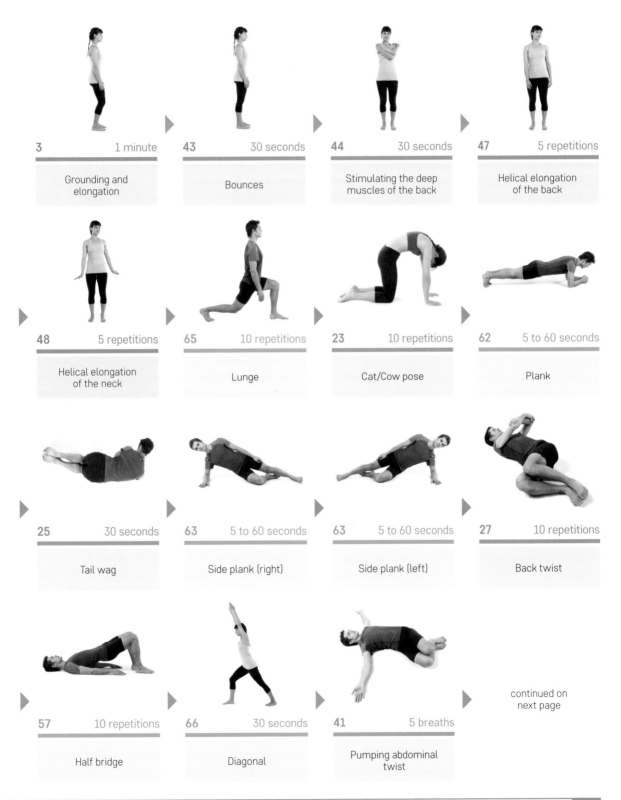

3   1 minute

Grounding and elongation

43   30 seconds

Bounces

44   30 seconds

Stimulating the deep muscles of the back

47   5 repetitions

Helical elongation of the back

48   5 repetitions

Helical elongation of the neck

65   10 repetitions

Lunge

23   10 repetitions

Cat/Cow pose

62   5 to 60 seconds

Plank

25   30 seconds

Tail wag

63   5 to 60 seconds

Side plank (right)

63   5 to 60 seconds

Side plank (left)

27   10 repetitions

Back twist

57   10 repetitions

Half bridge

66   30 seconds

Diagonal

41   5 breaths

Pumping abdominal twist

continued on next page

S3 Routine

Spinal 3 / 40 minutes (continued)
A full and varied routine for your back
▶ **Intermediate to advanced**
See Chapter 6 for more details on each numbered exercise.

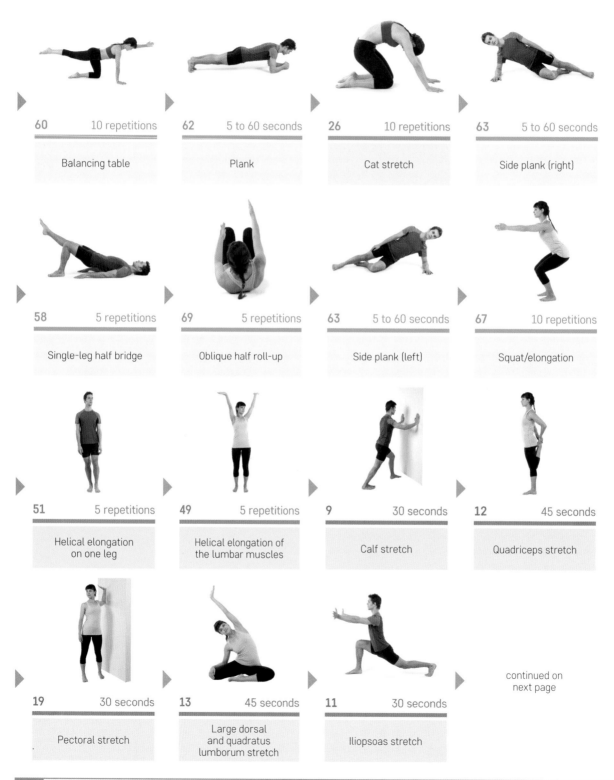

60 — 10 repetitions
Balancing table

62 — 5 to 60 seconds
Plank

26 — 10 repetitions
Cat stretch

63 — 5 to 60 seconds
Side plank (right)

58 — 5 repetitions
Single-leg half bridge

69 — 5 repetitions
Oblique half roll-up

63 — 5 to 60 seconds
Side plank (left)

67 — 10 repetitions
Squat/elongation

51 — 5 repetitions
Helical elongation on one leg

49 — 5 repetitions
Helical elongation of the lumbar muscles

9 — 30 seconds
Calf stretch

12 — 45 seconds
Quadriceps stretch

19 — 30 seconds
Pectoral stretch

13 — 45 seconds
Large dorsal and quadratus lumborum stretch

11 — 30 seconds
Iliopsoas stretch

continued on next page

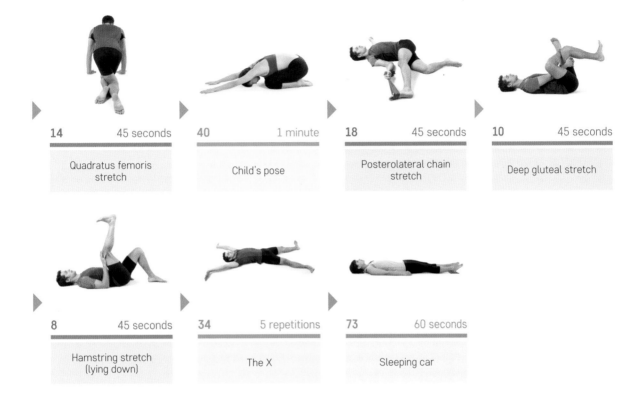

14	45 seconds

Quadratus femoris stretch

40	1 minute

Child's pose

18	45 seconds

Posterolateral chain stretch

10	45 seconds

Deep gluteal stretch

8	45 seconds

Hamstring stretch (lying down)

34	5 repetitions

The X

73	60 seconds

Sleeping car

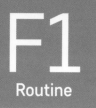

F1
Routine

Flex 1 / 5 minutes
More flexibility in just 5 minutes
▸ **For all**
See Chapter 6 for more details on each numbered exercise.

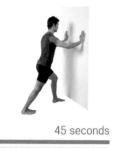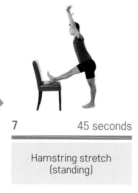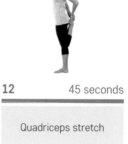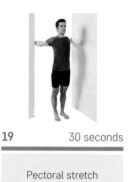

9 45 seconds	**7** 45 seconds	**12** 45 seconds	**19** 30 seconds
Calf stretch	Hamstring stretch (standing)	Quadriceps stretch	Pectoral stretch

F2
Routine

Flex 2 / 12 minutes
The main muscles you need to stretch
▸ **For all**
See Chapter 6 for more details on each numbered exercise.

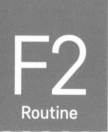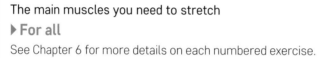

9 45 seconds	**7** 45 seconds	**12** 45 seconds	**19** 30 seconds
Calf stretch	Hamstring stretch (standing)	Quadriceps stretch	Pectoral stretch

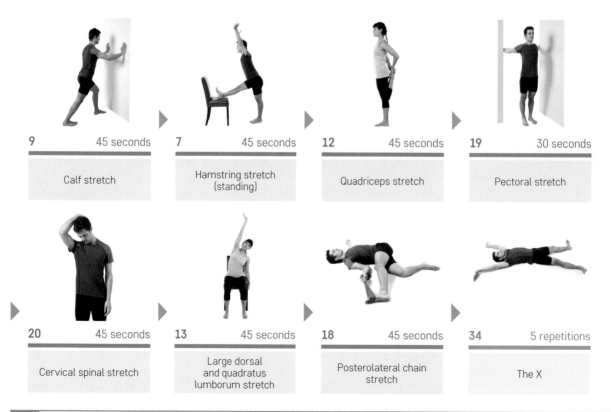

20 45 seconds	**13** 45 seconds	**18** 45 seconds	**34** 5 repetitions
Cervical spinal stretch	Large dorsal and quadratus lumborum stretch	Posterolateral chain stretch	The X

Flex 3 / 20 minutes
Full flexibility routine
For all ◀
See Chapter 6 for more details on each numbered exercise.

F3
Routine

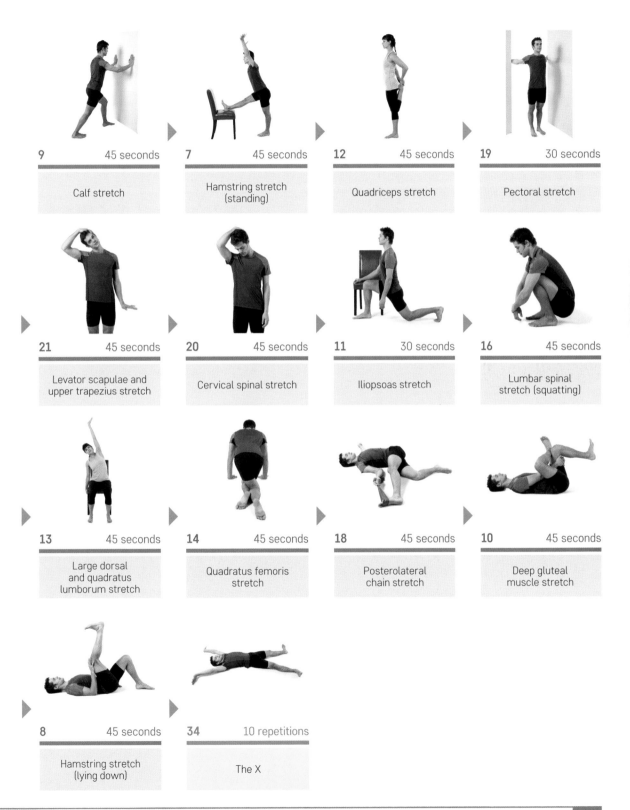

9 — 45 seconds
Calf stretch

7 — 45 seconds
Hamstring stretch (standing)

12 — 45 seconds
Quadriceps stretch

19 — 30 seconds
Pectoral stretch

21 — 45 seconds
Levator scapulae and upper trapezius stretch

20 — 45 seconds
Cervical spinal stretch

11 — 30 seconds
Iliopsoas stretch

16 — 45 seconds
Lumbar spinal stretch (squatting)

13 — 45 seconds
Large dorsal and quadratus lumborum stretch

14 — 45 seconds
Quadratus femoris stretch

18 — 45 seconds
Posterolateral chain stretch

10 — 45 seconds
Deep gluteal muscle stretch

8 — 45 seconds
Hamstring stretch (lying down)

34 — 10 repetitions
The X

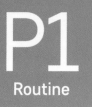

P1 Routine

Power 1 / 4 minutes
Activate your deep muscles in just a few minutes
▶ **Intermediate**
See Chapter 6 for more details on each numbered exercise.

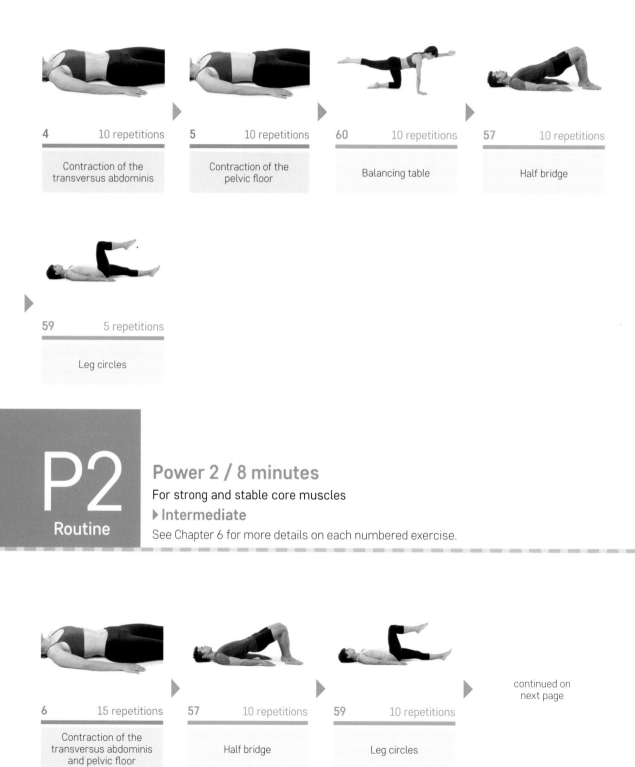

4 10 repetitions
Contraction of the transversus abdominis

5 10 repetitions
Contraction of the pelvic floor

60 10 repetitions
Balancing table

57 10 repetitions
Half bridge

59 5 repetitions
Leg circles

P2 Routine

Power 2 / 8 minutes
For strong and stable core muscles
▶ **Intermediate**
See Chapter 6 for more details on each numbered exercise.

6 15 repetitions
Contraction of the transversus abdominis and pelvic floor

57 10 repetitions
Half bridge

59 10 repetitions
Leg circles

continued on next page

Power 2 / 8 minutes (continued)
For strong and stable core muscles
Intermediate ◀
See Chapter 6 for more details on each numbered exercise.

P2
Routine

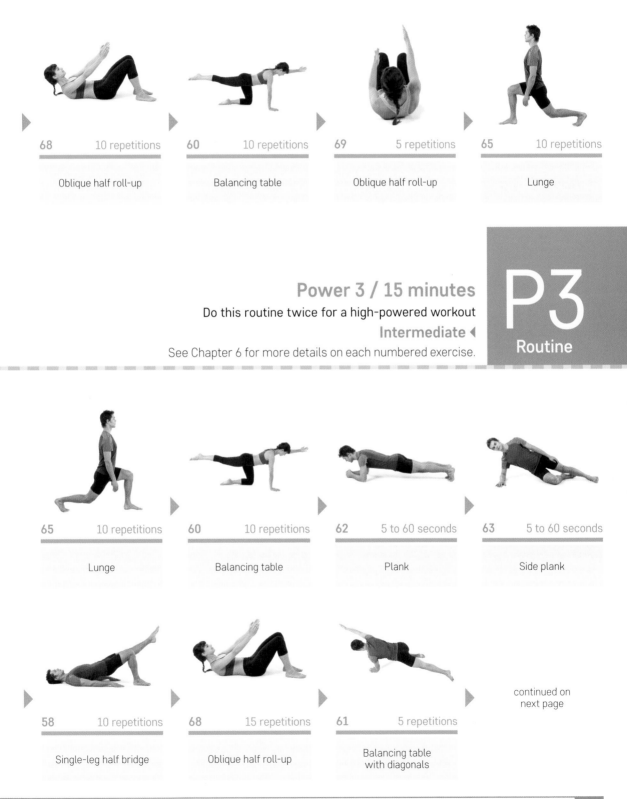

| **68** 10 repetitions | **60** 10 repetitions | **69** 5 repetitions | **65** 10 repetitions |
| Oblique half roll-up | Balancing table | Oblique half roll-up | Lunge |

Power 3 / 15 minutes
Do this routine twice for a high-powered workout
Intermediate ◀
See Chapter 6 for more details on each numbered exercise.

P3
Routine

| **65** 10 repetitions | **60** 10 repetitions | **62** 5 to 60 seconds | **63** 5 to 60 seconds |
| Lunge | Balancing table | Plank | Side plank |

| **58** 10 repetitions | **68** 15 repetitions | **61** 5 repetitions | continued on next page |
| Single-leg half bridge | Oblique half roll-up | Balancing table with diagonals | |

P3 Routine

Power 3 / 15 minutes (continued)
Do this routine twice for a high-powered workout
▶ Intermediate
See Chapter 6 for more details on each numbered exercise.

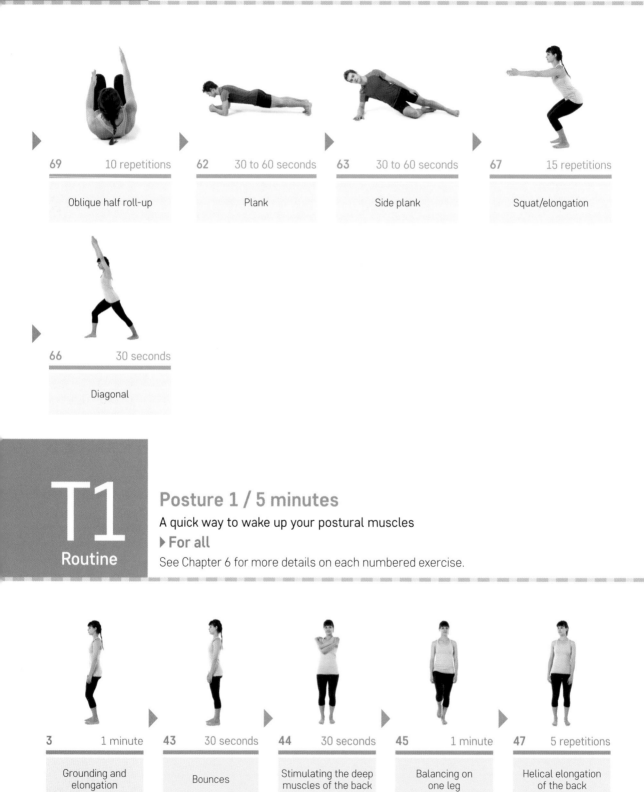

69 — 10 repetitions
Oblique half roll-up

62 — 30 to 60 seconds
Plank

63 — 30 to 60 seconds
Side plank

67 — 15 repetitions
Squat/elongation

66 — 30 seconds
Diagonal

T1 Routine

Posture 1 / 5 minutes
A quick way to wake up your postural muscles
▶ For all
See Chapter 6 for more details on each numbered exercise.

3 — 1 minute
Grounding and elongation

43 — 30 seconds
Bounces

44 — 30 seconds
Stimulating the deep muscles of the back

45 — 1 minute
Balancing on one leg

47 — 5 repetitions
Helical elongation of the back

Posture 2 / 12 minutes
To develop a new posture
For all ◄
See Chapter 6 for more details on each numbered exercise.

T2
Routine

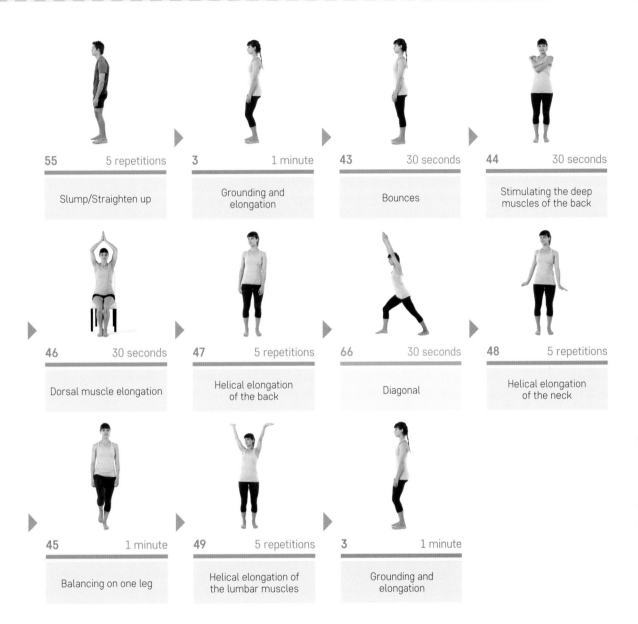

55 — 5 repetitions	**3** — 1 minute	**43** — 30 seconds	**44** — 30 seconds
Slump/Straighten up	Grounding and elongation	Bounces	Stimulating the deep muscles of the back
46 — 30 seconds	**47** — 5 repetitions	**66** — 30 seconds	**48** — 5 repetitions
Dorsal muscle elongation	Helical elongation of the back	Diagonal	Helical elongation of the neck
45 — 1 minute	**49** — 5 repetitions	**3** — 1 minute	
Balancing on one leg	Helical elongation of the lumbar muscles	Grounding and elongation	

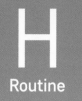

H
Routine

Helical / 8 minutes
A new way to stimulate the deep muscles of your back
▶ **For all**
See Chapter 6 for more details on each numbered exercise.

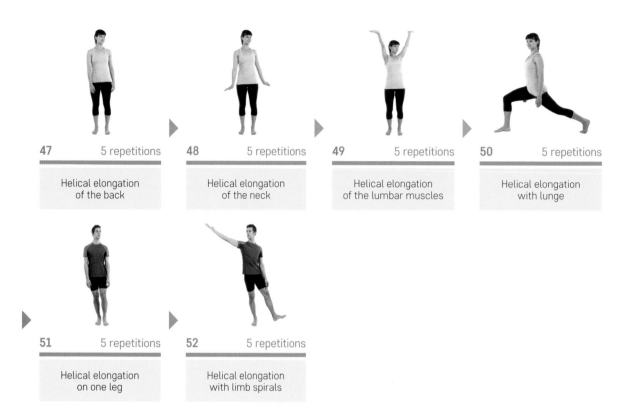

47   5 repetitions

Helical elongation
of the back

48   5 repetitions

Helical elongation
of the neck

49   5 repetitions

Helical elongation
of the lumbar muscles

50   5 repetitions

Helical elongation
with lunge

51   5 repetitions

Helical elongation
on one leg

52   5 repetitions

Helical elongation
with limb spirals

360° / 4 minutes per cycle

For strong and stable core muscles. Do one to four cycles

Intermediate to advanced ◀

See Chapter 6 for more details on each numbered exercise.

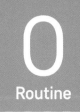

Routine

CYCLE 1

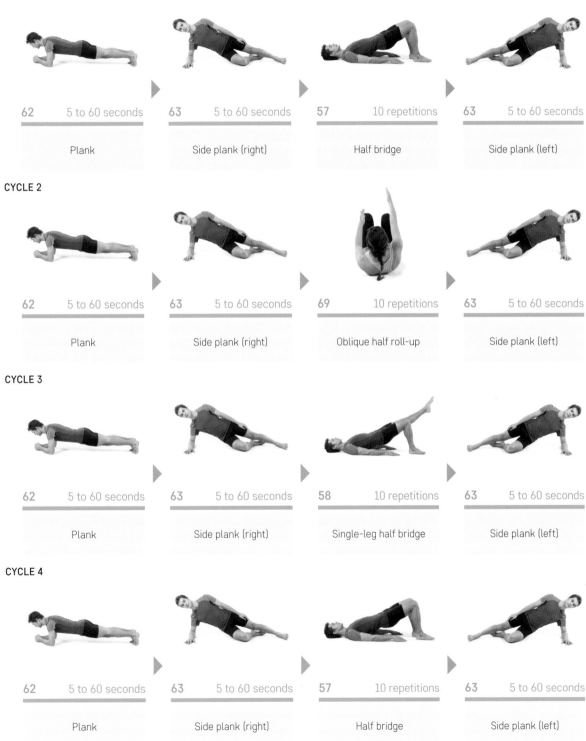

62	5 to 60 seconds	63	5 to 60 seconds	57	10 repetitions	63	5 to 60 seconds
Plank		Side plank (right)		Half bridge		Side plank (left)	

CYCLE 2

62	5 to 60 seconds	63	5 to 60 seconds	69	10 repetitions	63	5 to 60 seconds
Plank		Side plank (right)		Oblique half roll-up		Side plank (left)	

CYCLE 3

62	5 to 60 seconds	63	5 to 60 seconds	58	10 repetitions	63	5 to 60 seconds
Plank		Side plank (right)		Single-leg half bridge		Side plank (left)	

CYCLE 4

62	5 to 60 seconds	63	5 to 60 seconds	57	10 repetitions	63	5 to 60 seconds
Plank		Side plank (right)		Half bridge		Side plank (left)	

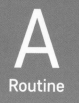
Awakening / 5 minutes

To start the day right

▶ **For all**

See Chapter 6 for more details on each numbered exercise.

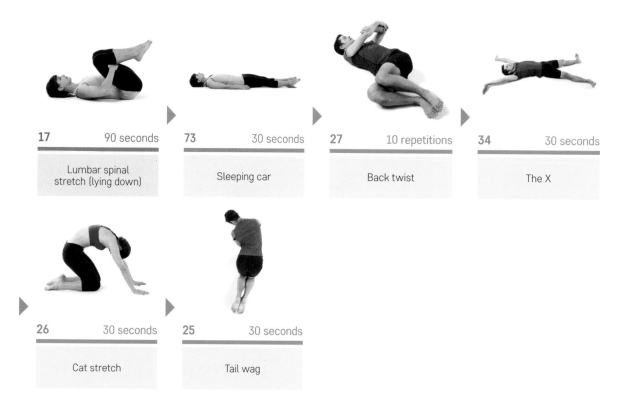

17 — 90 seconds
Lumbar spinal stretch (lying down)

73 — 30 seconds
Sleeping car

27 — 10 repetitions
Back twist

34 — 30 seconds
The X

26 — 30 seconds
Cat stretch

25 — 30 seconds
Tail wag

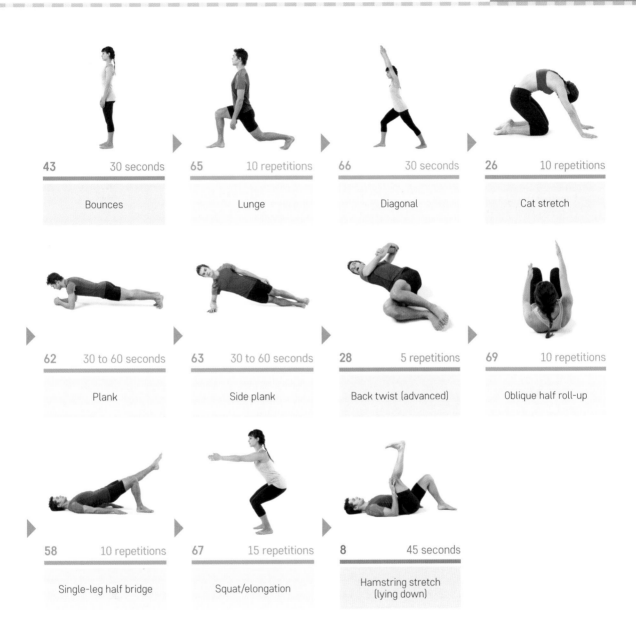

43   30 seconds

Bounces

65   10 repetitions

Lunge

66   30 seconds

Diagonal

26   10 repetitions

Cat stretch

62   30 to 60 seconds

Plank

63   30 to 60 seconds

Side plank

28   5 repetitions

Back twist (advanced)

69   10 repetitions

Oblique half roll-up

58   10 repetitions

Single-leg half bridge

67   15 repetitions

Squat/elongation

8   45 seconds

Hamstring stretch (lying down)

Intense 2 / 22 minutes

To energize your back

▶ **Intermediate to advanced**

See Chapter 6 for more details on each numbered exercise.

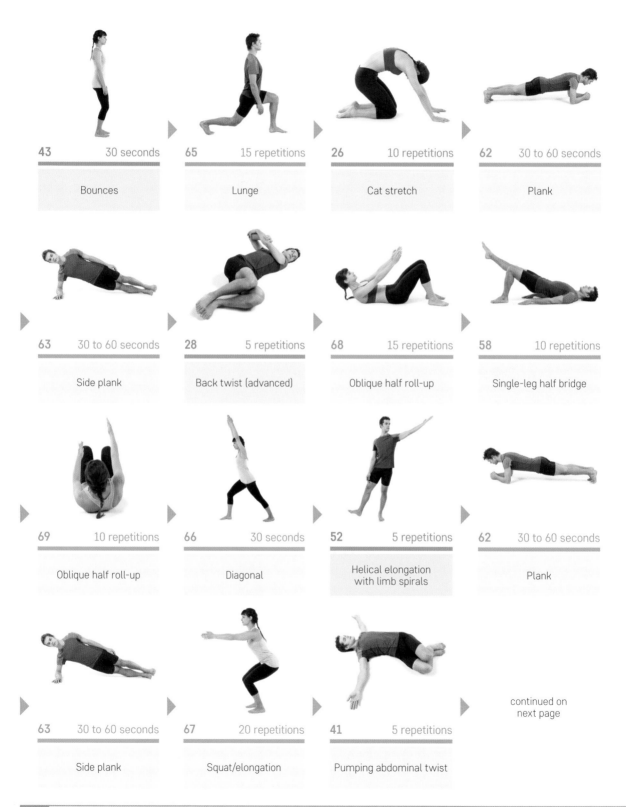

43	30 seconds	**65**	15 repetitions	**26**	10 repetitions	**62**	30 to 60 seconds
Bounces		Lunge		Cat stretch		Plank	

63	30 to 60 seconds	**28**	5 repetitions	**68**	15 repetitions	**58**	10 repetitions
Side plank		Back twist (advanced)		Oblique half roll-up		Single-leg half bridge	

69	10 repetitions	**66**	30 seconds	**52**	5 repetitions	**62**	30 to 60 seconds
Oblique half roll-up		Diagonal		Helical elongation with limb spirals		Plank	

63	30 to 60 seconds	**67**	20 repetitions	**41**	5 repetitions	
Side plank		Squat/elongation		Pumping abdominal twist		continued on next page

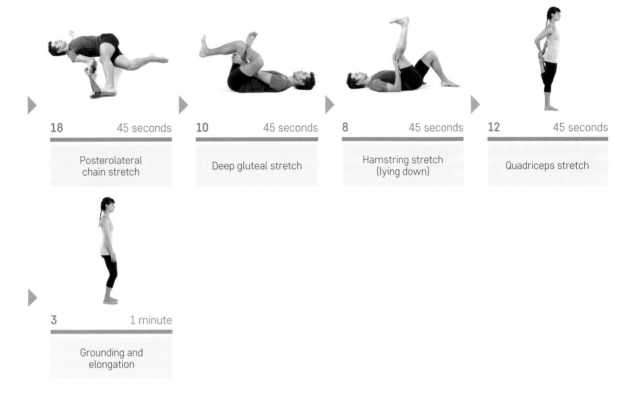

18   45 seconds

Posterolateral chain stretch

10   45 seconds

Deep gluteal stretch

8   45 seconds

Hamstring stretch (lying down)

12   45 seconds

Quadriceps stretch

3   1 minute

Grounding and elongation

Breathing / 12 minutes

Take the time to breathe and become more aware of your body

▶ **For all**

See Chapter 6 for more details on each numbered exercise.

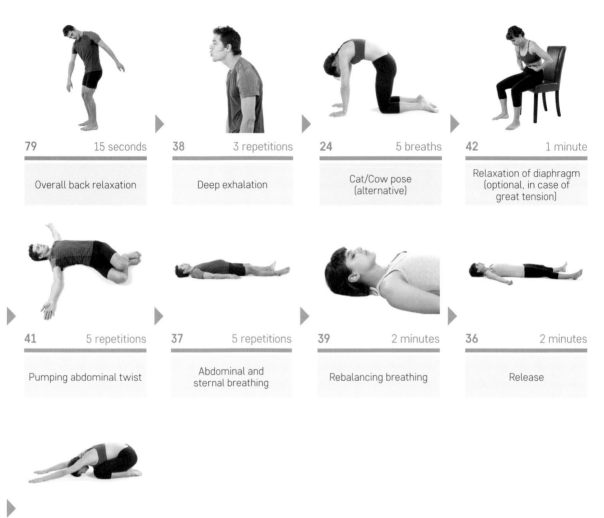

79 15 seconds	**38** 3 repetitions	**24** 5 breaths	**42** 1 minute
Overall back relaxation	Deep exhalation	Cat/Cow pose (alternative)	Relaxation of diaphragm (optional, in case of great tension)

41 5 repetitions	**37** 5 repetitions	**39** 2 minutes	**36** 2 minutes
Pumping abdominal twist	Abdominal and sternal breathing	Rebalancing breathing	Release

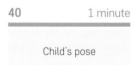

40 1 minute
Child's pose

Balance / 10 minutes

Mind and body feeling a little scattered? This routine is for you

For all ◀

See Chapter 6 for more details on each numbered exercise.

Y
Routine

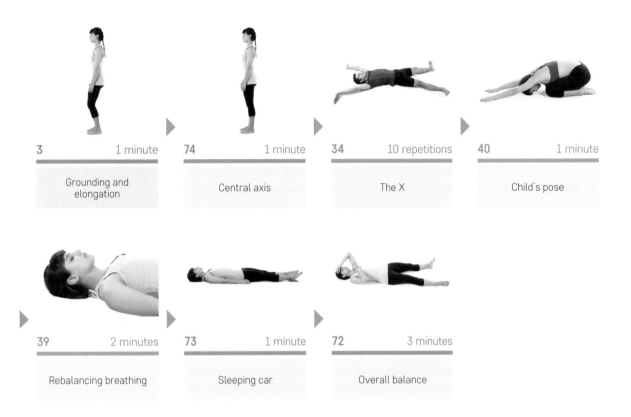

3   1 minute

Grounding and elongation

74   1 minute

Central axis

34   10 repetitions

The X

40   1 minute

Child's pose

39   2 minutes

Rebalancing breathing

73   1 minute

Sleeping car

72   3 minutes

Overall balance

Z1
Routine

Before bed 1 / 3 minutes
If you haven't moved all day and you're exhausted, try this routine
▶ **For all**
See Chapter 6 for more details on each numbered exercise.

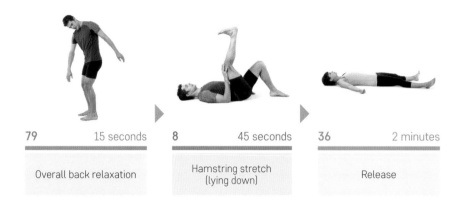

| **79** | 15 seconds | **8** | 45 seconds | **36** | 2 minutes |

| Overall back relaxation | Hamstring stretch (lying down) | Release |

Z2
Routine

Before bed 2 / 10 minutes
A great way to get your body ready for a good sleep
▶ **For all**
See Chapter 6 for more details on each numbered exercise.

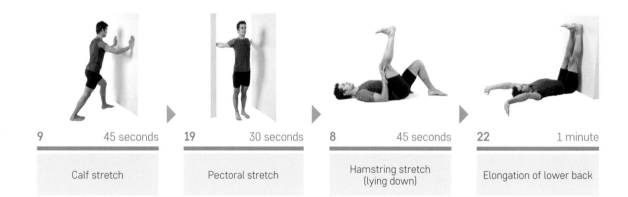

| **9** | 45 seconds | **19** | 30 seconds | **8** | 45 seconds | **22** | 1 minute |

| Calf stretch | Pectoral stretch | Hamstring stretch (lying down) | Elongation of lower back |

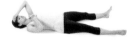

| **72** | 3 minutes |

| Overall balance |

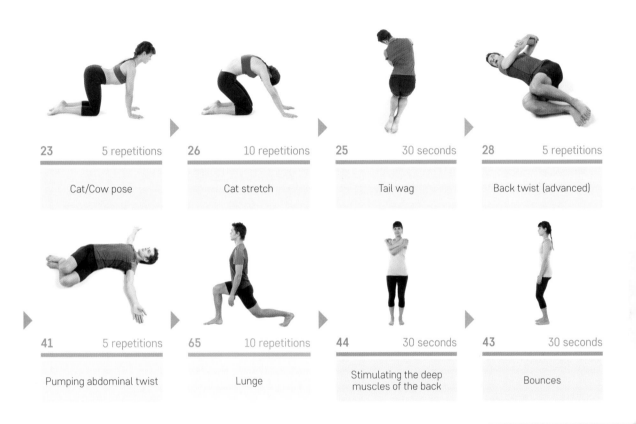

23 — 5 repetitions
Cat/Cow pose

26 — 10 repetitions
Cat stretch

25 — 30 seconds
Tail wag

28 — 5 repetitions
Back twist (advanced)

41 — 5 repetitions
Pumping abdominal twist

65 — 10 repetitions
Lunge

44 — 30 seconds
Stimulating the deep muscles of the back

43 — 30 seconds
Bounces

After a long walk 1 / 4 minutes
A few minutes to stretch the main areas that are tense after a walk

For all ◀

See Chapter 6 for more details on each numbered exercise.

W1
Routine

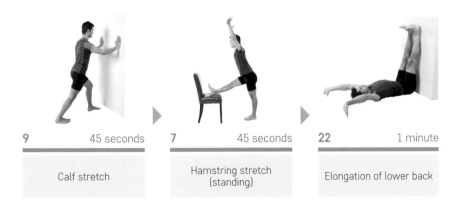

9 — 45 seconds
Calf stretch

7 — 45 seconds
Hamstring stretch (standing)

22 — 1 minute
Elongation of lower back

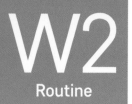

W2
Routine

After a long walk 2 / 8 minutes
For travelers and people who walk a lot
▶ For all
See Chapter 6 for more details on each numbered exercise.

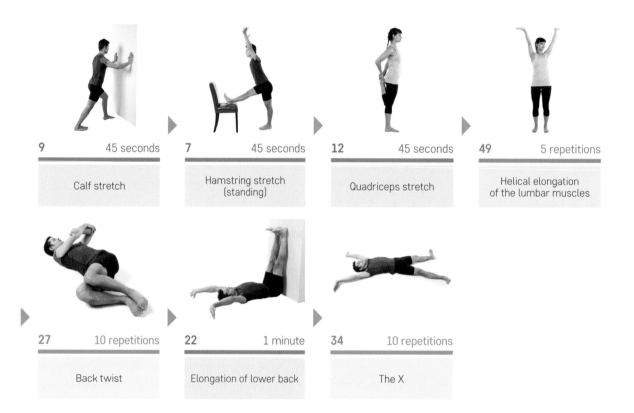

9   45 seconds
Calf stretch

7   45 seconds
Hamstring stretch (standing)

12   45 seconds
Quadriceps stretch

49   5 repetitions
Helical elongation of the lumbar muscles

27   10 repetitions
Back twist

22   1 minute
Elongation of lower back

34   10 repetitions
The X

Here are a few exercises that are great to do in the car, while keeping your eyes on the road, of course! Some exercises need to be adjusted for a seated posture

For all ◀

See Chapter 6 for more details on each numbered exercise.

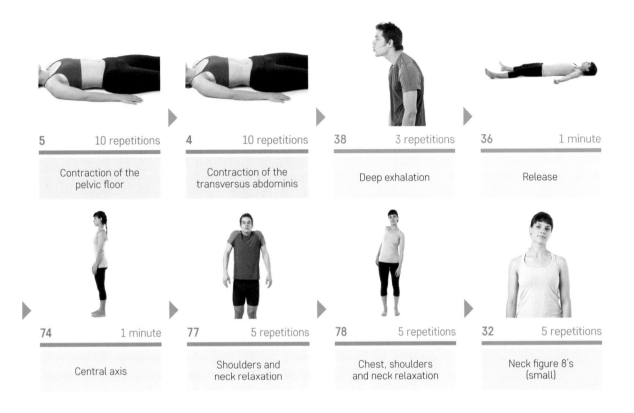

5 — 10 repetitions
Contraction of the pelvic floor

4 — 10 repetitions
Contraction of the transversus abdominis

38 — 3 repetitions
Deep exhalation

36 — 1 minute
Release

74 — 1 minute
Central axis

77 — 5 repetitions
Shoulders and neck relaxation

78 — 5 repetitions
Chest, shoulders and neck relaxation

32 — 5 repetitions
Neck figure 8's (small)

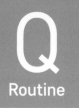
Computer

Do one of these exercises as a mini-break to avoid accumulating tension at the computer (at least every 60 minutes – ideally every 30 minutes)

▶ For all

See Chapter 6 for more details on each numbered exercise.

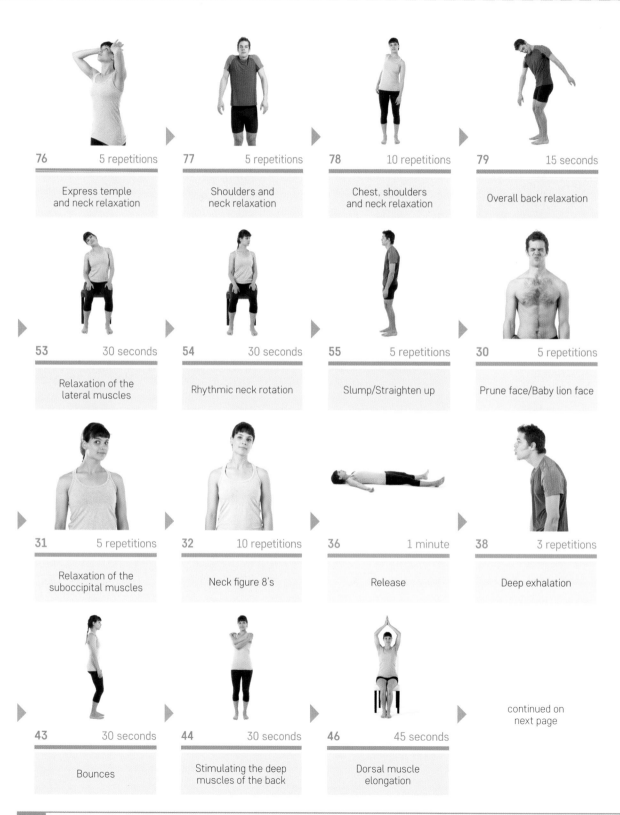

76 — 5 repetitions
Express temple and neck relaxation

77 — 5 repetitions
Shoulders and neck relaxation

78 — 10 repetitions
Chest, shoulders and neck relaxation

79 — 15 seconds
Overall back relaxation

53 — 30 seconds
Relaxation of the lateral muscles

54 — 30 seconds
Rhythmic neck rotation

55 — 5 repetitions
Slump/Straighten up

30 — 5 repetitions
Prune face/Baby lion face

31 — 5 repetitions
Relaxation of the suboccipital muscles

32 — 10 repetitions
Neck figure 8's

36 — 1 minute
Release

38 — 3 repetitions
Deep exhalation

43 — 30 seconds
Bounces

44 — 30 seconds
Stimulating the deep muscles of the back

46 — 45 seconds
Dorsal muscle elongation

continued on next page

Computer (continued)

Do one of these exercises as a mini-break to avoid accumulating tension at the computer (at least every 60 minutes – ideally every 30 minutes)

For all ◄

See Chapter 6 for more details on each numbered exercise.

Q
Routine

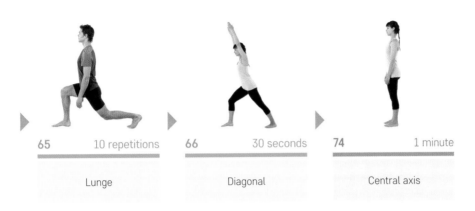

65	10 repetitions	66	30 seconds	74	1 minute
	Lunge		Diagonal		Central axis

Dorsal 1 / 4 minutes

A quick way to release the dorsal muscles and chest

For all ◄

See Chapter 6 for more details on each numbered exercise.

D1
Routine

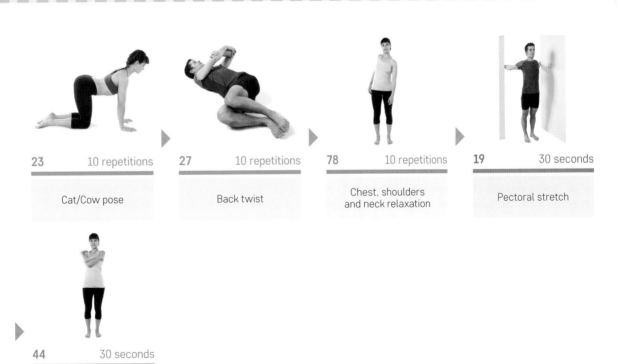

23	10 repetitions	27	10 repetitions	78	10 repetitions	19	30 seconds
	Cat/Cow pose		Back twist		Chest, shoulders and neck relaxation		Pectoral stretch

44   30 seconds

Stimulating the deep muscles of the back

Dorsal 2 / 12 minutes
To make your dorsal muscles and chest feel good
▶ **For all**
See Chapter 6 for more details on each numbered exercise.

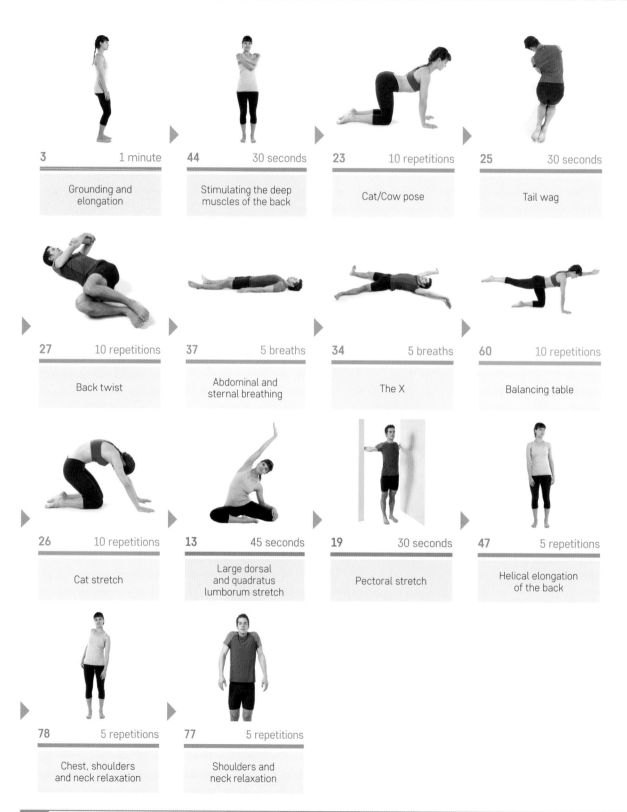

3 — 1 minute
Grounding and elongation

44 — 30 seconds
Stimulating the deep muscles of the back

23 — 10 repetitions
Cat/Cow pose

25 — 30 seconds
Tail wag

27 — 10 repetitions
Back twist

37 — 5 breaths
Abdominal and sternal breathing

34 — 5 breaths
The X

60 — 10 repetitions
Balancing table

26 — 10 repetitions
Cat stretch

13 — 45 seconds
Large dorsal and quadratus lumborum stretch

19 — 30 seconds
Pectoral stretch

47 — 5 repetitions
Helical elongation of the back

78 — 5 repetitions
Chest, shoulders and neck relaxation

77 — 5 repetitions
Shoulders and neck relaxation

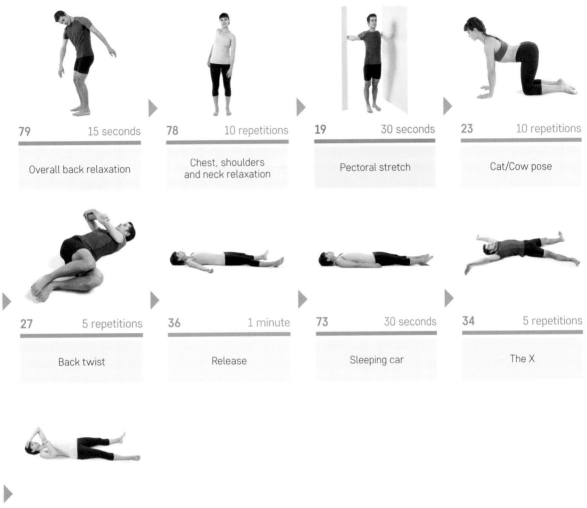

79 — 15 seconds
Overall back relaxation

78 — 10 repetitions
Chest, shoulders and neck relaxation

19 — 30 seconds
Pectoral stretch

23 — 10 repetitions
Cat/Cow pose

27 — 5 repetitions
Back twist

36 — 1 minute
Release

73 — 30 seconds
Sleeping car

34 — 5 repetitions
The X

72 — 3 minutes
Overall balance

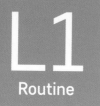

L1
Routine

Lumbar 1 / 5 minutes
Your lower back will feel better in just a few minutes
▶ **For all**
See Chapter 6 for more details on each numbered exercise.

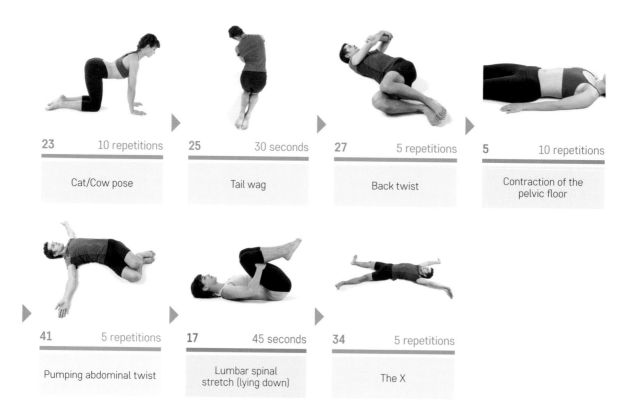

23 10 repetitions	**25** 30 seconds	**27** 5 repetitions	**5** 10 repetitions
Cat/Cow pose	Tail wag	Back twist	Contraction of the pelvic floor

41 5 repetitions	**17** 45 seconds	**34** 5 repetitions
Pumping abdominal twist	Lumbar spinal stretch (lying down)	The X

Lumbar 2 / 18 minutes
Keep lower back problems at bay
For all ◄
See Chapter 6 for more details on each numbered exercise.

L2
Routine

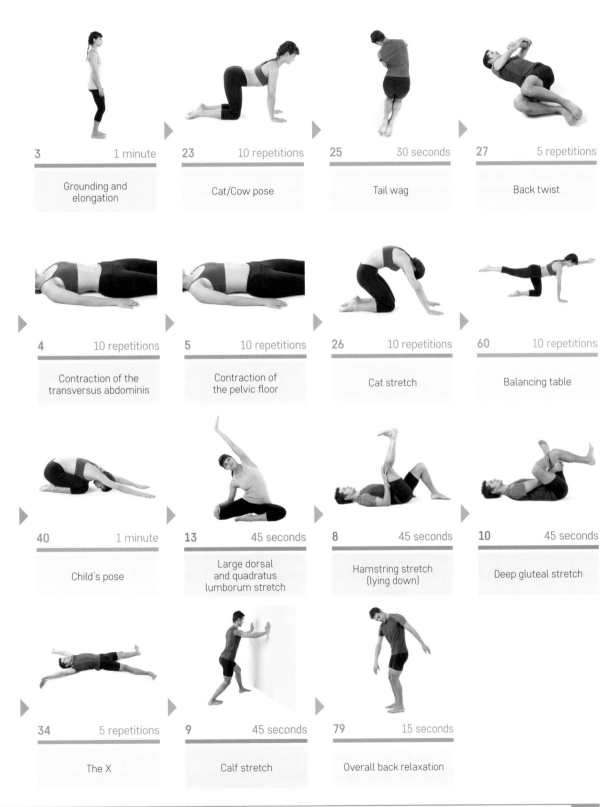

3	1 minute
Grounding and elongation	

23	10 repetitions
Cat/Cow pose	

25	30 seconds
Tail wag	

27	5 repetitions
Back twist	

4	10 repetitions
Contraction of the transversus abdominis	

5	10 repetitions
Contraction of the pelvic floor	

26	10 repetitions
Cat stretch	

60	10 repetitions
Balancing table	

40	1 minute
Child's pose	

13	45 seconds
Large dorsal and quadratus lumborum stretch	

8	45 seconds
Hamstring stretch (lying down)	

10	45 seconds
Deep gluteal stretch	

34	5 repetitions
The X	

9	45 seconds
Calf stretch	

79	15 seconds
Overall back relaxation	

Lumbar relief / 10 minutes

If your lower back is aching, do these exercises slowly

▶ **For all**

See Chapter 6 for more details on each numbered exercise.

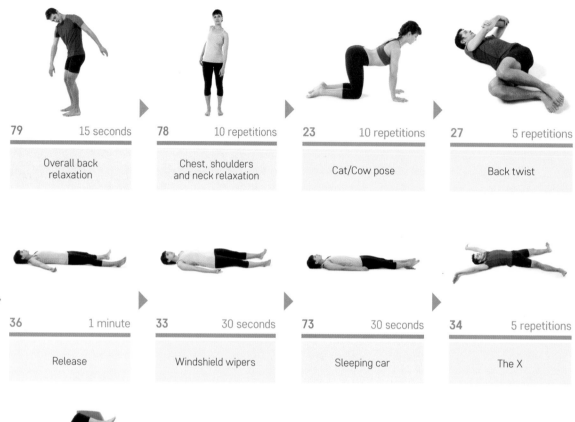

79   15 seconds

Overall back relaxation

78   10 repetitions

Chest, shoulders and neck relaxation

23   10 repetitions

Cat/Cow pose

27   5 repetitions

Back twist

36   1 minute

Release

33   30 seconds

Windshield wipers

73   30 seconds

Sleeping car

34   5 repetitions

The X

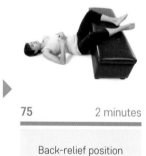

75   2 minutes

Back-relief position

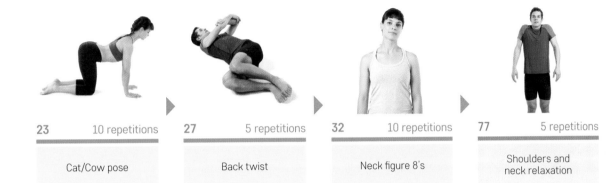

23 10 repetitions	**27** 5 repetitions	**32** 10 repetitions	**77** 5 repetitions
Cat/Cow pose	Back twist	Neck figure 8's	Shoulders and neck relaxation

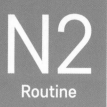

N2
Routine

Neck 2 / 10 minutes
Help for your fragile neck in just 10 minutes
▶ For all
See Chapter 6 for more details on each numbered exercise.

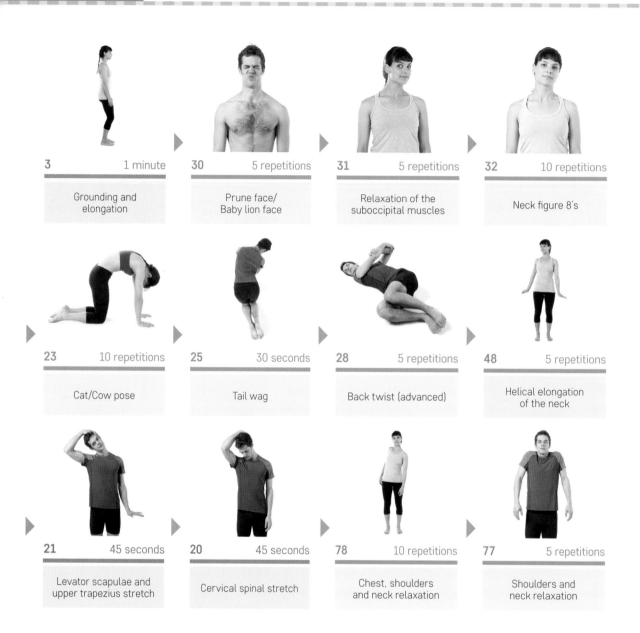

3 — 1 minute
Grounding and elongation

30 — 5 repetitions
Prune face/ Baby lion face

31 — 5 repetitions
Relaxation of the suboccipital muscles

32 — 10 repetitions
Neck figure 8's

23 — 10 repetitions
Cat/Cow pose

25 — 30 seconds
Tail wag

28 — 5 repetitions
Back twist (advanced)

48 — 5 repetitions
Helical elongation of the neck

21 — 45 seconds
Levator scapulae and upper trapezius stretch

20 — 45 seconds
Cervical spinal stretch

78 — 10 repetitions
Chest, shoulders and neck relaxation

77 — 5 repetitions
Shoulders and neck relaxation

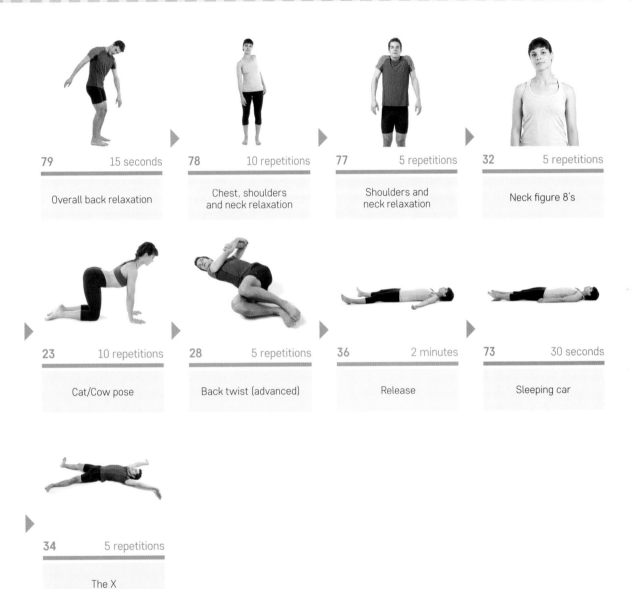

79	15 seconds	78	10 repetitions	77	5 repetitions	32	5 repetitions
Overall back relaxation		Chest, shoulders and neck relaxation		Shoulders and neck relaxation		Neck figure 8's	

23	10 repetitions	28	5 repetitions	36	2 minutes	73	30 seconds
Cat/Cow pose		Back twist (advanced)		Release		Sleeping car	

34	5 repetitions
The X	

Progressive
Program

This program is designed for those who want to slowly build up to a full training program for the back, one step at a time. Four weeks will give you time to master each exercise and gradually increase the duration and difficulty of your training. For details about each exercise, see Chapter 6.

Week 1

Objectives

- To learn the principles of elongation and grounding.
- To learn how to activate the core muscles.
- To mobilize the spinal column.

Day	Exercises	Duration of Routine
1	Elongation of the spinal column (1)	2 minutes
2	Elongation of the spinal column (1), Grounding (2)	4 minutes
3	Grounding and elongation (3)	2 minutes
4	Grounding and elongation (3), Contraction of the transversus abdominis (4)	4 minutes
5	Grounding and elongation (3), Contraction of the transversus abdominis (4), Contraction of the pelvic floor (5)	5 minutes
6	Cat/Cow pose (23), Contraction of the transversus abdominis and pelvic floor (6)	3 minutes
7	Cat/Cow pose (23), Contraction of the transversus abdominis and pelvic floor (6), Grounding and elongation (3)	5 minutes

Week 2

Objectives

- To learn the principles of flexibility exercises.
- To become aware of your breathing.
- To continue to improve mobility and posture.

Day	Exercises	Duration of Routine
8	Grounding and elongation (3), Contraction of the transversus abdominis and pelvic floor (6), Cat stretch (26)	4 minutes
9	Grounding and elongation (3), Contraction of the transversus abdominis and pelvic floor (6), Cat stretch (26), Back twist (27)	5 minutes
10	Contraction of the transversus abdominis and pelvic floor (6), Cat/Cow pose (23), Back twist (27), Calf stretch (9)	5 minutes
11	Cat stretch (26), Back twist (27), Calf stretch (9), Hamstring stretch (standing) (7), Grounding and elongation (3)	6 minutes
12	Cat/Cow pose (23), Back twist (27), Calf stretch (9), Hamstring stretch (standing) (7), Pectoral stretch (19), Grounding and elongation (3)	7 minutes
13	Release (36), Back twist (27), Cat/Cow pose (23), Cat stretch (26), Grounding and elongation (3)	8 minutes
14	Grounding and elongation (3), Cat stretch (26), Contraction of the transversus abdominis and pelvic floor (6), Back twist (27), Release (36), Calf stretch (9), Hamstring stretch (standing) (7), Pectoral stretch (19)	10 minutes

Week 3

Objectives
- To integrate the strengthening exercises.
- To master the helical elongations.
- To continue to improve on posture, flexibility and mobility.

Day	Exercises	Duration of Routine
15	Deep gluteal stretch (10), Back twist (27), Cat/Cow pose (23), Calf stretch (9), Hamstring stretch (standing) (7), Pectoral stretch (19), Grounding and elongation (3)	9 minutes
16	Tail wag (25), Cat stretch (26), Back twist (27), Deep gluteal stretch (10), Calf stretch (9), Hamstring stretch (standing) (7), Grounding and elongation (3)	9 minutes
17	Half bridge (57), Back twist (27), Release (36), Contraction of the transversus abdominis and pelvic floor (6), Deep gluteal stretch (10), Tail wag (25), Pectoral stretch (19)	10 minutes
18	Pumping abdominal twist (41), Cat/Cow pose (23), Tail wag (25), Half bridge (57), Deep gluteal stretch (10), Hamstring stretch (standing) (7), Grounding and elongation (3)	9 minutes
19	Helical elongation of the back (47), Cat stretch (26), Tail wag (25), Half bridge (57), Pumping abdominal twist (41), Calf stretch (9), Hamstring stretch (standing) (7), Pectoral stretch (19)	11 minutes
20	Grounding and elongation (3), Helical elongation of the back (47), Cat/Cow pose (23), Tail wag (25), Pumping abdominal twist (41), Half bridge (57), Calf stretch (9), Hamstring stretch (standing) (7), Pectoral stretch (19)	11 minutes
21	Grounding and elongation (3), Helical elongation of the back (47), Cat stretch (26), Tail wag (25), Back twist (27), Pumping abdominal twist (41), Half bridge (57), Deep gluteal stretch (10), Calf stretch (9), Hamstring stretch (standing) (7), Pectoral stretch (19)	13 minutes

Week 4

Objectives
- To emphasize the strengthening exercises.
- To continue to improve on posture, flexibility, mobility and breathing.

Day	Exercises	Duration of Routine
22	Grounding and elongation (3), Helical elongation of the back (47), Cat/Cow pose (23), Tail wag (25), Balancing table (60), Back twist (27), Pumping abdominal twist (41), Half bridge (57), Calf stretch (9), Hamstring stretch (standing) (7), Pectoral stretch (19)	13 minutes
23	Helical elongation of the back (47), Cat stretch (26), Tail wag (25), Balancing table (60), Pumping abdominal twist (41), Half bridge (57), Lunge (65), Calf stretch (9), Hamstring stretch (standing) (7), Pectoral stretch (19)	13 minutes
24	Grounding and elongation (3), Lunge (65), Cat/Cow pose (23), Balancing table (60), Back twist (27), Pumping abdominal twist (41), Half bridge (57), Large dorsal and quadratus lumborum stretch (13), Calf stretch (9), Hamstring stretch (standing) (7), Pectoral stretch (19)	14 minutes
25	Grounding and elongation (3), Cat/Cow pose (23), Tail wag (25), Balancing table (60), Back twist (27), Pumping abdominal twist (41), Plank (62), Deep gluteal stretch (10), Release (36), Large dorsal and quadratus lumborum stretch (13), Pectoral stretch (19)	14 minutes
26	Helical elongation of the back (47), Lunge (65), Cat stretch (26), Tail wag (25), Balancing table (60), Back twist (advanced) (27), Half bridge (57), Plank (62), Pumping abdominal twist (41), Deep gluteal stretch (10), Large dorsal and quadratus lumborum stretch (13), Hamstring stretch (standing) (7)	14 minutes
27	Helical elongation of the back (47), Lunge (65), Cat/Cow pose (23), Tail wag (25), Balancing table (60), Back twist (27), Half bridge (57), Pumping abdominal twist (41), Plank (62), Deep gluteal stretch (10), Hamstring stretch (lying down) (8), Large dorsal and quadratus lumborum stretch (13), Calf stretch (9), Pectoral stretch (19)	15 minutes
28	Grounding and elongation (3), Helical elongation of the back (47), Lunge (65), Cat stretch (26), Tail wag (25), Balancing table (60), Back twist (27), Pumping abdominal twist (41), Half bridge (57), Plank (62), Large dorsal and quadratus lumborum stretch (13), Hamstring stretch (lying down) (8), Calf stretch (9), Pectoral stretch (19)	15 minutes

Chart 24

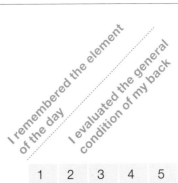

Day

I exercised my back

I remembered the element of the day

I evaluated the general condition of my back

1 = posture completely collapsed and very little energy

5 = good posture half the time with medium-level energy

10 = excellent posture and full of energy

	1	2	3	4	5	6	7	8	9	10

Day	Element										
24	Elongated spinal column										
23	String at the top of the skull										
22	Activated core muscles										
21	Sitting properly with neutral pelvis										
20	Jaw relaxed										
19	Walking with ease										
18	Breathing through abdomen										
17	Shoulders relaxed										
16	String at the top of the skull										
15	Neck elongated without effort										
14	Fluid spinal column										
13	Facial muscles relaxed										
12	Core muscles activated										
11	Keeping neck relaxed										
10	Legs solid and stable										
9	Head light and held high										
8	Properly seated on ischia										
7	Elongated spinal column										
6	Space between eyes relaxed										
5	Feet well grounded										
4	String at the top of the skull										
3	Breathing through abdomen										
2	Jaw relaxed										
1	Shoulders relaxed										

Note: In order to clearly see the steady progression of the state of your back, the chart has been devised in descending order of days, starting at Day 24 and going back to Day 1.

Acknowledgments

Many thanks to my associate editor, Élizabeth Paré, who was the best of collaborators. Thanks to her invaluable, committed and generous involvement, I was able to get through the writing process in the most wonderful way.

Thanks also to the entire editorial team, who guided me through the various stages of bringing this book to life.

Thanks to illustrator Chantale Boulianne for her unique artistic touch. She made *Homo sittingus* come to life.

Thanks to my team of trainers who helped me develop the Spinal Training Method. Émilie, Audrey and Emily, you are exceptional people and trainers.

Thanks to Emily Honegger, Audrey Lehouiller, Emmanuel Proulx and Simon Alarie who graciously consented to take part in the photo sessions.

Thanks to my esteemed professors, whose enthusiasm gave me the desire to pass on not only my knowledge but also a new way of seeing things.

Thanks to Philippe Druelle, osteopath, who instilled in me the very foundation that lies at the heart of this book: the body strives to be healthy.

Thanks to Jessica for your support and understanding.

Thanks to my parents who immersed me in a world of books and words and, in turn, gave me the desire to write a book.

References

Astin JA. *Mind-Body therapies for the management of pain. Clin J Pain*, 2004 Jan–Feb; 20 (1): 27–32.

Campignion, Philippe. *Les Chaînes Musculaires et Articulaires Concept GDS. Tome 1 Les Chaînes Antéro-latérales.* Philippe Campignion, 2004.

Clauzade Michel, and B. Darraillans. *Concept Ostéopathique de l'Occlusion.* Perpignan, S.E.O.O. 1989.

Courtois, Guy. *Neurologie.* Montréal: Les Presses de l'Université de Montréal, 1996.

Elkayam O., Ben Itzhak, S. et al. Multidisciplinary approach to chronic back pain: prognostic elements of the outcome. *Clin Exp Rheumatol*, 1996, May-Jun; 14 (3): 281-8.

Ernst, E. *The Complete Book of Symptoms and Treatments.* Massachusetts: Element Books Limited, 1998.

Gerard Tortora, and Sandra Reynolds Garbowski. *Principes d'Anatomie et de Physiologie,* Saint-Laurent, QC: ERPI, 2007.

Harvey J. and Wagner, P. *L'influence du Traitement Ostéopathique des Lésions non Physiologiques de la Colonne Vertébrale Sur le Test de Déhanchement,* 2006.

Kapandji Ibrahim Adalbert *Physiologie Articulaire.* Fascicule III, Sixième Édition. Paris: Maloine, 2007.

Korr Irvin. *Bases Physiologiques de l'Ostéopathie.* Paris: Frison-Roche, 1970.

Liebenson Craig. *Rehabilitation of the Spine: A Practitioner's Manual.* Philadelphia: Lippincott Williams & Wilkins, 2007.

Madignan L. et al. Management of symptomatic lumbar degenerative disk disease. *J Am Acad Orthop Surg,* 2009 Feb; 17(2): 102–111.

Magee David J. *L'Évaluation Clinique en Orthopédie.* Paris: Maloine, 1988.

Massion J. Postural control systems in developmental perspective. *Neurosci and Biobehav Rev,* 1998 Jul; 22 (4): 465–72.

McGill Stuart. *Low Back Disorders: Evidence-Based Prevention and Rehabilitation.* Illinois: Human Kinetics, 2007.

Mitchell Fred L., Jr. *The Muscle Energy Manual.* Vol. 3, Baltimore: MET Press, 1999.

Netter F. *Atlas d'Anatomie Humaine.* Masson (Educa Books), *2011.*

Page Phillip, Clare Frank and Robert Lardner. *Assessment and Treatment of Muscle Imbalance.* Illinois: Human Kinetics, 2010.

Richard Daniel and Didier Orsal. *Neurophysiologie.* Paris: Dunod, 2001.

Sasaki O, et al. Nonlinear analysis of orthostatic posture in patients with vertigo or balance disorders, *Neurosci Res,* 2001 Oct; 41 (2): 185–92.

Sibilia J., Pham T., Sordet C., et al. Spondylarthrite ankylosante et autres spondylarthrites, *EMC-Médecine,* 2005 Oct; Vol. 2, Issue 5: 488–511.

Statistics Canada. Canadian Community Health Survey. (ESCC3.1), 2005.

Statistics Canada. Adult Obesity in Canada: Measured Height and Weight. (ESCC3.1), 2008.

Tremblay M S, R C Colley, et al. Physiological and health implications of a sedentary lifestyle, *Appl Physiol Nutr Metab,* 2010 Dec; 35 (6): 725-40. doi: 10.1139/H10-079.

Struyf-Denys, Godelieve. *Les Chaînes Musculaires et Articulaires.* Bruxelles: ICTGDS, 1991.

Winter, DA. Human balance and posture control during standing and walking, *Gait & Posture,* 1995 Dec; Vol. 3, Issue 4. 193–214, 1995.

Woollacott M, et al. Neuromuscular control of the posture in the infant and child, *J Mot Behav,* 1987 Jun; 19(2): 167–86.

Woollacott M and A Shumway-Cook. Attention and the control of posture and gait: a review of an emerging area of research, *Gait Posture,* 2002 Aug; 16(1): 1–14.

World Health Organization. Low Back Pain, *Bulletin of the World Health Organization,* 2007.

Websites

Research chair on obesity, accessed November, 2010, www.obesite.ulaval.ca/obesite

Kino-Québec Science Committee (2008). Activité physique et santé osseuse [Physical Activity and Bone Health], http://www.kino-quebec.qc.ca/articles.asp, accessed December 2010

Ministère de l'Éducation, du Loisir et du Sport du Québec, accessed December, 2010, www.kino-quebec.qc.ca

National library of Medicine (Ed.). Pubmed, NCBI, accessed September, 2010, www.ncbi.nlm.nih.gov

World Health Organization. Physical inactivity: a global public health problem, accessed September, 2010, www.who.int/dietphysicalactivity/factsheet/inactivity

Index

joints, 76. *See also* mobility exercises

L

lateral muscles, 170
Leg Circles, 178
legs. *See also* hamstring muscles
  crossing, 57
  of unequal length, 37–38
levator scapulae stretches, 130
lifestyle, 30
load handling (lifting), 32, 40, 69
lumbago, 43
lumbar spine
  elongation of, 166
  routines for, 238–40
  stretches for, 124–26
Lunge, 167, 185
lungs, 34, 37. *See also* breathing; diaphragm

M

menopause, 35
mobility
  assessing, 100
  during cardio, 83
  exercises for, 76, 133–47, 165, 171
movement
  asymmetrical, 38, 39
  extreme, 71–72
  faulty, 31
  repetitive, 31, 39
muscles
  atonia in, 52
  of back, 24–25, 62, 63, 81
  imbalances in, 39
  phasic vs. tonic, 75
  strength assessment, 98
myths
  about abdominal muscles, 61, 79
  about fitness equipment, 69
  about floor exercises, 55
  about running, 83
  about standing up straight, 62
  about strengthening, 79, 81

N

neck
  elongation of, 59, 165
  eyes and, 55
  mobility exercises, 143–44, 165, 171
  pain in, 43
  relaxation exercises, 143, 199–203
  rotation of, 171
  routines for, 241–43
  stretches for, 129
  torticollis in, 46–47
nervous system, 76, 85. *See also* balance
Neuromuscular Relaxation, 202

O

obesity, 30–31
oblique muscles, 80
  exercises for, 189
oculomotor/oculocephalogyric reflex, 55
organs (internal), 34–35, 37
orthotics, 40
osteoarthritis, 30, 44, 45
osteoporosis, 45
Overall Balance, 194

P

pain. *See* back pain
pectoral stretches, 128
pelvic floor, 80
  exercises for, 112–13, 119, 190
pelvis, 57, 145. *See also* pelvic floor
  exercises for, 141, 191
piriformis muscle, 80
Plank
  front, 98, 182
  rotary (on wall), 184
  side, 183
  as strength assessment, 98
posterolateral chain stretches, 127
posture, 50–63
  assessing, 99
  during cardio, 83
  changing, 61–63
  effects, 31, 51
  exercises for, 77–78, 159–73
  mastering, 56–58
  muscle balance and, 39
power training, 81
premenstrual syndrome (PMS), 35
presbyopia, 36
progressive lenses, 36, 55
proprioceptors, 52–55
  exercises for, 185

Prune Face, 142
Pumping Abdominal Twist, 156

Q

quadratus femoris stretches, 122
quadratus lumborum muscle, 79, 80, 122
quadriceps stretches, 121

R

Reach for the Sky, 147
reconnection routine, 89–90
rectus abdominis muscle, 80
relaxation (of muscles), 62, 63. *See also*
   tension
   assessing, 99
   of back, 198
   during cardio, 83
   of chest, 157, 201
   exercises for, 194–203
   of lateral muscles, 170
   of neck, 143, 199–203
   in reconnection routine, 89–90
   of shoulders, 200–201
   during stretching, 115
Release, 150
resistance training, 81
rheumatoid polyarthritis, 44
Roll-Ups, 188–89
Rotary Plank on Wall, 184
running, 83

S

scars, 36–37
sciatic neuralgia/neuritis (sciatica), 43
scoliosis, 38
sedentary behavior, 17–21
shoes, 40, 56–57. *See also* feet
shoulder relaxation, 200–201
sitting. *See also* chairs
   ergonomics and, 62–63
   positions for, 57–58
   as posture assessment, 99
   problems caused by, 18–21
sit-ups, 11, 79
Sleeping Car, 196
slumping, 52, 172
smoking, 30
soleus stretches, 118

spinal column, 22–23. *See also* central axis;
   vertebrae
   curves in, 61
   disk problems, 32, 43–44
   elongation of, 59–61, 108, 110, 164, 173, 187
   location in body, 60
   organ problems and, 34
   as proprioceptor, 53
Spinal Training, 73. *See also* Spinal Training
   exercises
   breaks from, 94–95
   components, 75–85
   obstacles to, 89–91
   parameters, 74
   success tips, 92–95
Spinal Training exercises. *See also* Spinal
   Training routines
   for balance, 183–203
   basic, 107–13
   for breathing, 149–57
   for flexibility, 115–31
   for mobility, 133–47
   for posture, 159–73
   for strengthening, 175–91
Spinal Training routines, 207–9
   After a Long Walk (W), 231–32
   Awakening (A), 224
   Balance (Y), 229
   Before Bed (Z), 230
   Breathing (B), 228
   Car (K), 233
   Computer (Q), 234-35
   Dorsal (D), 235–37
   energizing, 225–27
   Flex (F), 216–17
   Helical (H), 222
   Intense (I), 225–27
   Lumbar (L), 238–40
   Neck (N), 241–43
   Posture (T), 220–21
   Power (P), 218–20
   Pre-cardio (V), 231
   Progressive Program, 208, 244–49
   Spinal (S), 210–15
   360° (O), 223
spondylolysis, 46
sports, 38
sprains, 43
Squat
   as exercise, 125, 187
   as strength assessment, 98

Library and Archives Canada Cataloguing in Publication

Harvey, Jean-François, 1973–
[Entraînement spinal. English]
  Cure back pain : 80 personalized easy exercises for spinal training to improve posture, eliminate tension & reduce stress / Jean-François Harvey, BSc, DO.

Includes index.
Translation of: L'entraînement spinal.
ISBN 978-0-7788-0531-1 (paperback)

  1. Backache—Exercise therapy. 2. Back exercises. I. Title. II. Title: Entraînement spinal. English.

RD771.B217H3713 2016   617.5'64062   C2015-908239-0